pn
10/5/06

REMAKING SOCIAL WORK WITH CHILDREN AND FAMILIES

Remaking Social Work with Children and Families provides a sustained examination of the 'modernisation' of this area of social care. It analyses some of the key themes introduced by the administrations of John Major and Tony Blair and provides a critical exploration of contemporary policy initiatives. These include:

- the *Looking after Children (LAC)* materials
- the *Framework for the Assessment of Children in Need and their Families*
- 'working together' to protect children
- the mainstream approach to 'race' and ethnicity in social work with children
- the relocation of adoption at the heart of social work
- the implications for social work of the emergence of 'personal advisers', mentors and related professionals.

The author argues that political and ideological factors need to be taken into account if we are to understand the dominant discourses and evolving ways of working with children and their families. Political fixation with ensuring that young people are able to 'fit' into their allotted roles in a market economy and an overarching concern about children and criminality have been crucial in this respect. He concludes that while social workers and educators should be prepared to embrace change, they need to be critical agents in the process of change, recognising the ever-present need to promote and foster democracy within the sphere of social welfare.

This timely book will be helpful to all students, educators and social care professionals who are seeking to develop their theoretical and practical understanding of a changing profession.

Paul Michael Garrett is a Senior Lecturer in Social Work at the University of Nottingham.

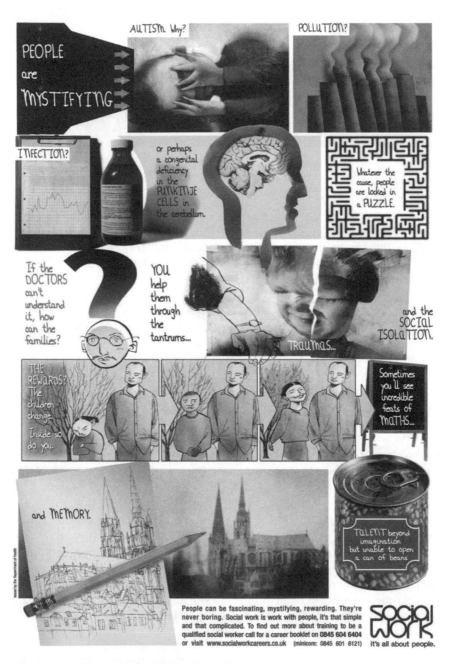

Autism – an advert from the Social Worker Recruitment Campaign

REMAKING SOCIAL WORK WITH CHILDREN AND FAMILIES

A critical discussion on the 'modernisation' of social care

Paul Michael Garrett

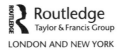

Routledge
Taylor & Francis Group

LONDON AND NEW YORK

First published 2003 by Routledge
11 New Fetter Lane, London EC4P 4EE

Simultaneously published in the USA and Canada
by Routledge
29 West 35th Street, New York, NW 10001

Routledge is an imprint of the Taylor & Francis Group

© 2003 Paul Michael Garrett

Typeset in Times by
BC Typesetting, Bristol
Printed and bound in Great Britain by
TJ International, Padstow, Cornwall

British Library Cataloguing in Publication Data
A catalogue record for this book is available from the British Library

Library of Congress Cataloging in Publication Data
Garrett, Paul Michael, 1958–
Remaking social work with children and families: a critical discussion
on the 'modernisation' of social care/Paul Michael Garrett.
p.   cm.
Includes bibliographical references and index.
ISBN 0-415-29836-9 – ISBN 0-415-29839-3 (pbk.)
1. Social work with children–Great Britain.
2. Child Welfare–Great Britain. 3. Family social work–Great Britain.
I. Title.
HV751.A6G37 2003
362.7′0941–dc21   2003043198

ISBN 0-415-29839-3 (pb)
ISBN 0-415-29836-9 (hb)

For Ciaran and Geileis, *Sonas agus Solas*

CONTENTS

ACKNOWLEDGEMENTS

A number of individuals have provided me with support and encouragement and should be warmly thanked. These include Paula Brady, Jill Anderson, Alan and Meryl Aldridge. Gerry Hanlon also read and commented on an earlier draft of Chapter 3 and Tim Strangleman did the same with Chapter 4. The social workers and police officers, whose comments form the core of the latter chapter, need to be thanked for finding the time to be interviewed by me. Edwina Welham, Michelle Bacca and Jamie Hood at Taylor & Francis provided welcome assistance and quickly answered my numerous queries. Alison Pilnick, Jose Lopez and Tony Fitzpatrick helpfully responded to my occasional state of puzzlement about the production of a book.

Some of the chapters in this book have appeared, in radically different form, as articles in academic journals or papers given at conferences. I remain, therefore, grateful for the suggestions of editors, referees and conference attendees for prompting me to ponder, in greater detail, some of the key themes and preoccupations which form the core of *Remaking Social Work with Children and Families*. An earlier version of Chapter 2 appeared in the Oxford University Press publication, the *British Journal of Social Work*, in 1999. Similarly, a different version of Chapter 4 appeared in the same journal in 2002. Earlier versions of Chapters 6 and 8 appeared in the Sage journal *Critical Social Policy* in 2002. In this context, I remain particularly grateful to Mark Drakeford and Ian Butler, the editors of the *British Journal of Social Work* and to the Editorial Collective of *Critical Social Policy*. Her Majesty's Stationery Office (HMSO) granted permission for me to reproduce Figure 1. It was originally published in Department of Health, Department for Education and Employment, Home Office, *Framework for the Assessment of Children in Need and their Families* (2000). Caroline Munkenbeck, Marketing Communications Manager, at the Department of Health provided permission for me to use one of the adverts, used during the social work recruitment campaign, for the frontispiece of the book.

Chapter 7 incorporates ideas featured in two papers: 'Neglecting Irish Children? Notes on Irish Children in Public Care in Britain and the Failure of Theory, Policy and Practice', which I gave at the annual general meeting of the All-Party Irish in Britain Parliamentary Group at the House of Commons in January 2001. This chapter also includes some of the thoughts included in another paper, 'Social Care Provision and Irish People in Britain: the Case of Social Work and Irish Children', which was delivered at the Renville Institute at the University of Helsinki in May 2002. I am grateful to John McDonnell MP and Pirkko Hautamäki for their invitations to write and present these papers. I, however, am entirely responsible for any errors, or shortcomings, which readers may detect in the book.

LIST OF ABBREVIATIONS

AAR	Action and Assessment Record
BASW	British Association of Social Workers
CAR	Core Assessment Record
CCETSW	Central Council for Education and Training in Social Work
COS	Charity Organisation Society
CS	Connexions Service
CSCI	Commission for Social Care Inspection
DfEE	Department for Education and Employment
DoH	Department of Health
DipSW	Diploma in Social Work
GSCC	General Social Care Council
ICS	Integrated Children's System
LAC	*Looking after Children: Assessing Outcomes in Children Care.* Also, and more frequently referred to, as the Looking after Children system
NCSC	National Care Standards Commission
PA	Personal Adviser
PIU	Performance Innovation Unit
QP	Quality Protects
SCIE	Social Care Institute for Excellence
SSD	Social Services Department
TOPSS	Training Organisation for Personal Social Services
YOT	Youth Offending Team
YJB	Youth Justice Board

1

INTRODUCTION

Thinking critically about social work with children and families in the early twenty-first century

In Britain, being asked to describe the shape of social work with children and families presents an immensely difficult task. In the early twenty-first century, on account of the bewildering rapidity of change in this particular sector of social care, it is almost like being asked to describe the finer detail of a speeding motorway driver's wristwatch whilst stood in an adjacent field. None the less, this book will attempt to provide a series of critical snapshots of key features of contemporary social work with children and families.[1]

Currently, this area of social work can be associated with a range of dominant preoccupations. These include:

- The fragmentation of local authority social work and the creation of new organisational forms of intervention in the lives of children and their families (e.g. the Sure Start initiative, Youth Offending Teams, the Connexions agency, etc.). Changes are also taking place across the adult and community care sector (see, for example, the editorial 'Under health, by stealth', *Community Care*, 8–14 November 2001: 5).
- The proliferation of 'performance targets', 'outcome' measures and other types of quantitative data demanded by the New Labour administration (Ward and Skuse 2001; see also Clarke and Newman 1997; Newman 2001; Arkin 2001; Travers 2001). Related to this has been the introduction into practice of a plethora of centrally devised 'tools', which have had an impact on the *process* of social work with children and families.
- An emphasis on agencies 'working together' and 'joined up' approaches.
- A renewed emphasis on the centrality of child adoption, particularly as an option for children who are in public care, or 'looked after' under the Children Act 1989.
- Poor morale and a staffing recruitment crisis. Only 4,703 people applied to the social work admissions system for courses starting in 2001

compared with 11,526 in 1995: a fall of 59 per cent (see the editorial 'A boost for students', *Community Care*, 3–9 October 2002: 5). This crisis prompted, in 2001–2, in a series of advertisements in the national press (Department of Health 2001a; Unison 2002).

• The publication of National Occupation Standards and reorganisation of social work education (Orme 2001).

• The introduction of a new regulatory structure for social work and social care. Related to this has been the installation of a new, or reconfigured, panoply of quangos and 'alphabet agencies', including the General Social Care Council (GSCC), the Training Organisation for Personal Social Services (TOPSS), Social Care Institute for Excellence (SCIE), the National Care Standards Commission (NCSC) and, more recently, the Commission for Social Care Inspection (CSCI).

• The continuing public inquiry examining the circumstances relating to the death of Victoria Climbié (Department of Health 2001b). Furthermore, there is, of course, speculation about the impact of the inquiry on child protection services (Association of Directors of Social Services 2002a; Kendall and Harker 2002; Local Government Association, NHS Confederation, Association of Directors of Social Services 2002). In the early twenty-first century, concerns were also expressed about social work responses to other children – including Chelsea Brown, Ainlee Labonte and Lauren Wright – who were killed by their carers.

Clearly, this list is not exhaustive and some of the preoccupations and themes relate to social work, in general, and not simply to social work with children and families. It might also be suggested that some of these developments are situated in a wider public domain (for example, the Climbié case) whilst others (for example, the increasing use of centrally devised 'tools' for practice) are, perhaps, of interest and concern only to social workers and related staff. None the less, at the time of writing, these remain some of the main issues and they will provide part of the substance of the book, or part of the backdrop for the ensuing discussion.

A central contention in this book is that we are witnessing the *remaking* of social work with children and families. Furthermore, the focal aim will be to critically analyse this process. In short, how did social work with children and families come to look the way that it does in the early twenty-first century? What assessments, moreover, are we able to make about its future trajectory and shape? The intention will not be to try and mount a reactive defence of 'old' ways of working or anachronistic organisational forms. There can, for example, be no going back to the social work of the pre-Thatcherite period and to the economic and social circumstances which gave rise to the particular character of social work then. This is not a volume that nostalgically yearns for a return to a 'Golden Age' of pure and benevolent social work endeavour (see, in this context,

Strangleman 1999). Moreover, there will be no forsaken attempt to represent social work as an entirely benign – or 'empowering' activity – which has become freshly contaminated by political and managerial imperatives.

In examining the remaking of social work with children and families, the book's focus will largely be on local authority social work in England and Wales. It is, however, suggested that developments here are apt to have implications for social work theory and practice elsewhere in Europe and even farther afield. Indeed, the 'ways of seeing' social work being promoted here – and the operational modalities which these visions give rise to – tend to lead to changes to social work processes in other national settings. For example, cultural artefacts (the plethora of protocols, schedules and assessment 'tools' devised in England) frequently become exports. Furthermore, the export potential of the various 'systems' and 'frameworks' for social work and social welfare is enhanced in the context of more embracing global transformations (Pugh and Gould 2000; see also Jameson 2000; Mann 2001). Important here is also the fact that the new states comprising the former Eastern Bloc are frequently seeking to model theory and practice on British and American approaches (Iarskaia-Smirnova and Romanov 2002).[2] The materials associated with the influential *Looking after Children: Assessing Outcomes in Child Care* project (LAC), for example, are now being deployed amongst, we are advised, 'Aboriginal peoples in Western Australia and the Inuit of Labrador' as well as being used with children and families in Canada, Sweden, Hungary and Russia (Ward 2000b: 134; see also Parker *et al.* 1991; Gray 2002: 193–4). In brief, some of the issues at the heart of this book, although relating to social work in Britain, will have resonance across national boundaries.

The fluidity and ambiguity of 'social work'

As an activity 'social work' is, of course, socially constructed and culturally and historically unstable (see also International Federation of Social Workers 2000). Consequently, changes in the modalities of social work intervention, reflected in, for example, the LAC system and the *Framework for the Assessment of Children in Need and their Families* should not surprise (Department of Health, Department for Education and Employment, Home Office 2000).[3] Bar-on (1999: 9), for example, in his discussion on the development of social work in Africa, points out that social work training in Botswana originally took place in 'an agricultural college where students were taught 'cooking, knitting, vegetable gardening and the like'. In short, the activity constructed and identified as 'social work' – here entirely abstracted from, for example, a preoccupation with 'frameworks' and schedules – was partly shaped and determined by the context in which it took place and evolved.

In a European context, however, Zygmunt Bauman (2000a), commenting on the 'proceduralisation' of social work, evidenced by the increased use of centrally devised schedules and 'instruments', has expressed concern that 'daily practice' is becoming 'ever more distant from its original ethical purpose' (Bauman 2000a: 9). He reminds his readers that 'social work, whatever else it may be, is also the ethical gesture of taking responsibility for the fate and well-being of the Other' (Bauman 2000a: 10). He goes on:

> Clarity and unambiguity may be the ideal of the world in which 'procedural execution' is the rule. For the ethical world, however, ambivalence and uncertainty are the daily bread and cannot be stamped out without destroying the moral substance of responsibility, the foundation on which the world rests.

In a humanistic sense, therefore, this tension between the 'original ethical impulse' and 'procedural execution' might be viewed as the focal point for a range of dilemmas which confront social workers, particularly in a context where – as we shall see – micro-engagements with the users of services are increasing being plotted by centrally devised assessment schedules and measured by quantitative performance indicators. Nonetheless, it could be countered that Bauman's magisterial overview, although welcome because his comments run counter to the hegemony of managerialism and the practitioner cynicism it is apt to engender inside welfare bureaucracies, is not entirely convincing on account of the way he perceives the 'original' ethical purpose of social work.

In Britain, it could be argued that the motivations, impulses and preoccupations of the Charity Organisation Society (COS), the forerunner of modern social work, were more complex than his analysis would suggest (see Jones 1983). To be sure, there was a concern *about* 'the Other', but how the recipients of services were constructed – in the language of the day as the 'industrial residuum' (Dendy 1895) – suggests a project far less benign and more regulatory and disciplinary. From these early days, social work interventions were intent on reinforcing *particular* economic and gender relations. Even during this early period, marking the beginning of professional social work, there was also an early fixation with proceduralisation (see Richmond 1917). Furthermore, this understanding also relates to the notion that 'British child welfare practice has suffered from a lack of historical reflection' (Stevenson 1998: 154). Indeed, perhaps social work needs to be more attentive to the historical dimension.[4] Clearly if there is a failure to interrogate the collective professional past, social work will be ill equipped to analyse and respond to more contemporary 'blueprints' for practice such as the highly influential LAC system.

Reviewing the radical critique(s)

In Britain, in the late 1970s, many social work academics and practitioners did begin to re-examine social work's role in society and the way in which it functioned. Central here was an emerging recognition that the tasks of social workers could only be properly understood in the context of the political economy. A range of 'radical' texts, therefore, identified social work as part of the capitalist state's ideological apparatus (Simpkin 1983; see also Althusser 1971). These contributions remain insightful, but the more vulgar variants of Marxism were, perhaps, too economically reductive and insufficiently attentive to structural discrimination and oppression also rooted in racism (Dominelli 1988) and patriarchy (Kemp and Squires 1997). More recently, within social work, there have been attempts to evolve more inclusive counter-discourses and strategies and these can be associated with 'anti-discriminatory practice', 'anti-racist practice' and 'anti-oppressive practice'.

All these ideas did not, however, evolve in a social and economic vacuum, but were a by-product of the struggles, throughout civil society and stretching back into the late 1960s, of a range of social movements which had alternative visions of how the world might be organised (Harman 1988). Contestations, taking place in the industrial West and elsewhere included: a reinvigorated struggle, partly informed by Marxism, but also more libertarian currents, for workers' rights and industrial democracy (Meiksins Wood 1995); the battle for women's equality (Segal 1987; Brah 1992: 34–40) and for gay liberation (Segal 1990: ch. 6); the fight for racial equality in the metropolitan centres and for national self-determination for 'subordinate' nations confronted by imperialism and neo-colonialism (Dooley 1998). This period also witnessed the birth of an inchoate 'politics of disability' (Oliver 1984) and a mental health system 'survivors' movement (see Rogers and Pilgrim 1989).

Another critique of the idea that social work is a deeply ethical – even liberatory or 'empowering' – activity has, more recently, been provided by those influenced by post-structuralism and particularly Foucault (1977; see also Rojek 1986; Webb and McBeath 1989; Parton 1991; Rodger 1991). This approach perceives social work as one facet of 'disciplinary power' which Foucault associated with the evolution of the 'psy professions' (psychology, psychiatry, criminology) and the spread of new discourses and technologies of treatment and surveillance (see also Donzelot 1979; Cohen 1979, 1985; Rose 1985, 1989). During the 1990s, the related social theory of postmodernism also had some impact on social work theorising (see McBeath and Webb 1991; Nuccio and Sands 1992; Gorman 1993; Howe 1994; Pardeck et al. 1994; Parton 1994; Pozatek 1994; Parton and Marshall 1998; Pease and Fook 1999; Fawcett et al. 2000; see also Carter 1998). However, social work's belated postmodernist turn had little real impact on field social work, as perceived by its practitioners. Perhaps more fundamentally, the more 'extreme' or 'sceptical' postmodernist orientations have been cogently criticised from *within* social work (Peile and McCourt 1997; Smith and White 1997; Ferguson and Lavalette 1999; Williams 1999).[5]

'No space of innocence'? Governmentality and social work

The contribution of Foucault remains significant for those trying to grasp the meaning and intent of social work. For him, 'government' needed to be conceived in the broad way in which it was viewed in the sixteenth century. During that period 'government', therefore, did:

> not simply refer to political structures or the management of states; rather it designated the way in which the conduct of individuals or states might be directed: the government of children, of souls, of communities, of families, of the sick . . . It did not cover only the legitimately constituted forms of political or economic subjection . . . To govern, in this sense, is to structure the possible fields of action.
>
> (Foucault in Harris 1999: 30; see also Rose 1996: 38; Dean 1999)

Foucault's contribution and the subsequent literature influenced by it can, therefore, be viewed as helpfully expanding our understanding of what constitutes ruling and 'governance' (see also Rose 1998: 10–18). This conceptualisation and its 'analytics of government' would perceive social work as complicit in the strategies of governance (Johnson 1993) – part of the assemblage of micro-practices which comprise contemporary modes of government (see also Fraser 1989: 17–35).

The autonomy of experts and expertise is, however, important for governmentality theorists. Rose and Miller (1992: 180), for example, argue that 'Liberal government identifies a domain outside of "politics" and seeks to manage it without destroying its autonomy.' This is made possible through the 'activities and calculations of a proliferation of independent agents' including social policy formulators and practitioners, such as social workers. Here, 'political forces' seek to 'utilise, instrumentalise and mobilise techniques and agents other than those of "the state" in order to "govern at a distance"' (Rose and Miller 1992: 181). However, experts and expertise – embodying neutrality, authority and skill – fulfil a crucial role because they 'hold out the hope that the problems of regulation can remove themselves from the disputed terrain of politics and relocate into the tranquil seductive territory of truth' (Rose and Miller 1992: 188).

More recently, Rose (1993: 285) in articulating the concept of 'advanced liberal rule' has stressed the relocation of experts within a 'market governed by the rationalities of competition, accountability and consumer demand' (see also Rose 1996: 40–1). It might, of course, be countered that expertise and experts are no longer, in a 'risk society', unquestionably accepted as possessing unimpeachable attributes of authority and skill (see Beck 1998). However, Rose (1993: 295) has, in part, acknowledged this shift in that his conceptualisation of 'advanced liberal rule' recognises the 'dialectic of hope and suspicion today attached to experts and their truths'. For him, this development can be associated with a 'reconfiguration of the political salience of expertise' and 'a new way of "responsibilizing" experts in relation to claims made upon them other than those of their own criteria of truth and competence' (Rose 1996: 55). A number of writers, not associated with the governmentality approach, have also looked at changes taking place with regard to the professions and professional identities. Some have specifically examined the implications of 'responsibilising' for the welfare professions as a whole (Foster and Wilding 2000; Malin 2000), or particular fields of welfare, such as probation (Nellis 1999; Robinson 2001; Sparrow et al. 2002).

Importantly, those influenced by the governmentality literature exhibit a certain pessimism. Despite the claims of 'radical social work' throughout the late 1970s and early 1980s (Jones 1983), Amy Rossiter (2000: 32), a social work academic based in Canada, has argued that there is no 'space of innocence' which permits the choice of being 'an agent of social change or being an agent of social control' (Rossiter 2000: 32). Problems are further compounded because social work has 'barely begun the work of understanding its construction within power' (emphasis added). Hence it continues to seek to rely on 'notions of innocent helping to legitimate its presence'. However, for her, there is 'no help . . . outside of governmentality'.

Having accepted that the governmentality literature helps to promote new insights, it is, therefore, also important to recognise that there are problems associated with this conceptual approach. Fitzpatrick (2002: 14) has asserted that the theorists of governmentality resemble 'foreign correspondents' who are reporting, but 'unwilling to intervene'. On account of this orientation, the 'dispossessed' are likely to regard 'post-structuralist non-intervention as affluent self-indulgence' (see also Harris 1999: 27). More fundamentally, because of an antipathy for anything resembling 'meta-histories of promise' and a preference for 'militancy grounded in scholarly moderation', some of the leading intellectual interventions associated with governmentality theory appear to rule out the possibility of human agency and fail to appreciate the significance of counter-discourses and oppositional practices (see, particularly, Dean 1999: ch. 3).

The notion of 'governing at a distance' and expert autonomy is perhaps questionable when applied to local authority social work, in Britain. As we shall see, throughout the 1990s and early twenty-first century, there have been concerted attempts to render social work – the 'invisible trade' (Pithouse 1998) – more visible and less autonomous. Furthermore, as the

7

LAC system, the Framework and the whole 'competences' approach central to social work education indicate, social work – not only with children and families, but more generally – has become more industrialised, with centrally devised modalities being used to 'Taylorize the labour process and impose technological controls over the work' (Dominelli and Hoogvelt 1996: 55; see also Fabricant 1985).[6]

The approach adopted in the book

This book is not intent on providing an 'alternative vision' of the future of social work with children and families in Britain. The more limited intention will be examine the remaking of this aspect of social work by interrogating a number of its dominant, or 'official', discourses. What, for example, does 'working together' actually amount to in terms of the working relationships between social workers and police officers in the context of the child protection endeavour? How might we interpret and try to understand some of the key ideas that are at the heart of the LAC system? How might we regard the current political and professional fixation with the adoption of children? How do more abstract ideas about 'work' and 'criminality' impact on social work with children and families? In relation to 'race' and ethnicity, is social work's tendency to view the world in binary terms – or 'black' and 'white' – obscuring identity issues for many children and families? In brief, parts of the book will seek to provide critical interpretations of some of child-care social work's organising themes.

As well as providing a searching examination of these dominant discourses, the book will also try to 'move in closer' and investigate a number of key modalities of social work intervention. More specifically, the aim will be to narrow the focus and to direct our lens at some of the recently introduced 'tools' for social work practice with children and families. This is because, as Janet Newman (2001: 146) has argued, it is important in all fields of social welfare to stress the way in which discourses do 'not operate merely at the level of language and culture, but are also embedded in technologies and practices'. Aspects of the political agenda of New Labour, for example, include trying to alter the vocabulary and ideology previously central to the discourse on the welfare state in Britain (Fairclough 2000). How, for example, is this translated into the technologies and practices being promoted by the *Framework for the Assessment of Children in Need and their Families* (Department of Health, Department for Education and Employment, Home Office 2000)?

Part of the argument developed in the book is that if we are to examine the remaking of social work with children and families we need, therefore, to do more than have regard to the big themes and leading discourses. We also need to scrutinise the emerging technologies and material practices of social work. The proliferation of centrally devised assessment schedules which social workers are compelled to use in their daily encounters with children and families – such as the LAC system and the Framework – are rarely critically investigated, yet they provide a basis for examining the changing character of social work. Forms can, of course, be viewed as 'humble and mundane mechanisms' (Rose and Miller 1992: 183), mere adjuncts to the core activity of social welfare practice. However, the approach to be developed here shares an interpretation which suggests that 'prescriptive and proscriptive documents are a form of organisational governance' (Taylor and White 2000: 149). More specifically, the materials discussed later help to illuminate how social workers are being shaped and regulated and how an arid approach to the *work* in social work risks being promoted (see also Gubruim *et al.* 1989). Furthermore, these forms indicate how the users of services are fixed and processed. As Carolyn Taylor and Sue White (2000: 151) observe:

> Forms demand of their completers a description, not an argument, a debate or range of opinion. They demand that completers put aside doubts they may have about what they describe . . . and just get on with ticking the box and fixing the description. Once fixed as words or numbers these completed forms become data; they become fixed (in this context, also see Leonard 2000: 94).

What do the new forms and associated policy papers, featured so prominently in social work with children and families, reveal about the changes taking place? What does this documentation tell us about the shape or trajectory of social work in a new century? How is the activity of the social worker regulated and controlled? What does a close reading of these materials tell us about dominant perceptions of the users of services? What do mere sets of forms reveal about the remaking of social work and more rooted political concerns about, for example, 'troublesome' children? It will be argued that a detailed deconstruction of official, Department of Health (DoH) materials can, perhaps, provide insights into all these questions.

'Dolphins' and 'sharks': the critical ethic underpinning the book

The introduction of the Assessment Framework can be seen in terms of a journey that needs to be made by the workforce between the 'island of current assessment practice' and the 'island of new assessment practice' . . . The sharks can be seen as the . . . barriers to the introduction of change. The dolphins are the promoters of change.
(Department of Health, NSPCC, University of Sheffield 2000: 75)

This book, using some of the imagery associated with the new Framework materials, is, if not swimming *with* the dolphins, then swimming *alongside* them. That is to say, there is a recognition that there *should* be concern about the calibre or – in the dismal managerialist lexicon – the 'quality' of social work available for children and families.[7] As illustrated by the tragic case of Victoria Climbié, public perception of the role of social workers, in Britain, has, for example, been shaped by inquiries into the deaths of children which, albeit filtered by the media, have appeared to highlight a manifest lack of 'expertise' and 'professionalism' (see also London Borough of Brent 1985; London Borough of Greenwich 1987; London Borough of Lambeth 1987; Secretary of State for Social Services 1988; Sinclair and Bullock 2002). Revelations about the institutional abuse of children have had a further impact on the public perception of social work and social workers (Secretary of State for Health 1998a). Consequently, despite acknowledging the relative 'success' of, for example, child protection services in Britain (ADSS 2002a: 9), it will not be suggested in this book that previous ways of engaging with the users of services was satisfactory and that practitioners and social work academics should be complacent and inert.

Furthermore, social work is vulnerable to the assertion that there should be greater direction from the centre: that there needs to be, for example, a whole series of protocols, frameworks and schedules available to guide practitioners and to protect the public from poor, arbitrary, damaging or dangerous interventions. Moreover, it might be argued that there is nothing terribly wrong with standardisation and proceduralisation if consistent and transparent social work practice is being fostered and promoted. More fundamentally, social work should not be viewed as an 'exercise of internally regulated professionalism, answerable only to itself' (Lorenz 1994: 9). These arguments are compelling, but the book will also remain sensitive to the fact that the history of child welfare reform is ordinarily 'written simply as progressive narrative' and 'interrogative questions appear ungracious' (Hendrick 1994: preface). More fundamentally, perhaps at the risk of being daubed with the Blairite epithet 'wrecker', 'interrogative questions' will be posed, dissent will be shown, and a critical ethic will underpin the ensuing discussion.[8]

In addition, it is also important to be alert to the admonishment of Chris Jones (2001: 550) that 'so few people within social work seem to be talking or writing about' the changes taking place in relation to local authority social work. Surveying a 'traumatised, even defeated occupation which has lost any sense of itself', he has gone on to condemn 'the silence of the commentators, especially in the academy', for failing to investigate and report what is taking place on social work's 'front line'; a 'front line' staffed, moreover, by a largely female work force (Department of Health 2002a; see also 'Exodus of "worn-out" staff from public jobs', *The Guardian*,

3 September 2002; 'High anxiety and stacks of back-covering forms', *The Guardian*, 27 November 2002). This book will try, therefore, to remain mindful of the charge that there is now an immense cleavage separating the perceptions, interests and preoccupations of the mainstream (and expanding) social work academy from those actually doing the job. It will also attempt to provide critical insights, which take into account the *work*, which is at the heart of contemporary social work with children and families. In this sense the perspective to be developed here is also informed by the other contributions which have endeavoured to describe the changing contours of work in the late twentieth and early twenty-first centuries (see, for example, Casey 1995; Sennett 1999; Reich 2001; Cameron *et al.* 2002).

What follows is not an objective account, or *the* true account, of the remaking of social work with children and families. Furthermore, it is not being implied that writing from within a university facilitates revelatory insights. The higher education sector does not exist *outside* neo-liberalism and *apart* from the processes which are shaping other parts of the public sector. Indeed, it might be argued that many of the so-called 'top' universities in Britain, aping private corporations and heavy with a sense of their own worth and sense of importance, are increasingly beginning to inhabit a peculiar 'looking glass world' where some vice-chancellors can lobby for the introduction of 'top-up' fees to 'widen access' for the poorest (see also Harvie 2000). The aim is this book is merely to try and unsettle dominant and 'official' accounts, or discourses, and to generate a sense of 'epistemic reflexivity' (White in Taylor and White 2000: 35). The authorial aspiration is, therefore, to promote constructive criticism, but to avoid wanton, or capricious, polemic (see, in this context, Bauman 2000b; Bennett 1998: introduction). What this book does, however, accept is that child welfare, like other fields of the welfare, is an arena of struggle and contestation

The organisation of the book

In order to provide narrative impetus, the rest of the book will be organised in a loosely chronological way and will chart some of the key developments since the early 1990s. This is not, of course, to argue that prior to then social work with children and families was static and not subject to changes in theory and practice (see, for example, Parton 1991). More precisely, there is no implicit denial here of the devastating impact of the Thatcher years on civil society and the public services. However, beginning in the early 1990s provides a convenient route into some of the book's main themes. 1990 saw John Major succeed Margaret Thatcher as Prime Minister. Somewhat symbolically, as the year drew to a close, it also witnessed the death of Frederic Seebohm, whose report, in 1968, led to the creation of Social Services Departments (SSDs). The following year also saw the introduction – in October 1991 – of the Children Act 1989 and that same year the publication of the foundation text of the LAC system (Parker *et al.* 1991).

Both parts of the book, one largely dealing with the Major period and the other with the Blair administrations, will commence with a short preamble, which provides contextual information for some of the issues to be examined in greater detail. Part I will begin by exploring the LAC system which has been used – to varying degrees – by local authority Social Services Departments since the early 1990s. Whilst acknowledging the need for reforming how social workers assessed and related to 'looked after' children and young people, the chapter will illuminate problems, ambiguities and contradictions associated with the 'parenting' construct which lies at the heart of the scheme. It will then go on to discuss how the scheme relates to 'troublesome' children (Newburn 1996). This will include a detailed exploration of Action and Assessment Records (AARs) the main component of the LAC system (Ward 1995c). Here, it will be maintained that the AARs are potentially oppressive and contain powerful subtexts about, for example, 'appropriate' youth lifestyles and the nature of 'work'. Concerns are also expressed about how AARs risk being used as aids to facilitate the surveillance, screening and profiling of this group of young people (see also James and James 2001).

Chapter 3 will argue that the heavily promoted LAC project continues to exert a powerful influence on social work with children and families in Britain and elsewhere. Despite the repeated assertions that the documentation associated with LAC is embedded in 'objective' research, it is maintained that this is not sustainable on account of the failure of the scheme's designers to interrogate their own normative assumptions and judgements. In addition, it is asserted that the LAC project should be politically situated with the researchers' relationship with the Department of Health needing to be more fully explored.

Still concerned with developments during the period of Conservative hegemony, Chapter 4 will shift focus to examine a component of the 'working together' paradigm central to child protection since the 1980s. The inquiry into the death of Victoria Climbié has already highlighted how social workers, police officers and health professionals failed to 'work together' to protect the child. In this chapter the specific focus is on the social work/police relationship because – historically – this is where difficulties and ruptures have been most apparent (e.g. Cleveland, Rochdale, Nottingham, the Orkneys). Moreover, it is suggested that joint working between social workers and police officers needs to be properly examined because of the creation of multidisciplinary Youth Offending Teams (YOTs) and a more embracing preoccupation with 'joined up' approaches to child welfare services. Here, we will focus on interviews with social workers and police officers, which shed light on how they view and perceive their roles. Research discussed in this chapter will examine joint police/social work specialist units and it will be argued that here there is a troubling blurring of occupational roles and professional identities with social workers apt to be rendered subservient to the police.

Part II will investigate a number of the transformations that have occurred during the Blair period (Department of Health 1998d; see also Powell 1999). Here, it will be maintained that, in terms of social work with children and families, there are continuities with the Major period (graphically represented by how the Framework builds on the LAC materials), but also significant differences. Chapter 5 will examine this Framework which is the first 'official' standard assessment model intended for use in the initial assessment of all 'children in need' under Part 111, section 17 of the Children Act 1989. Here it is argued that this new 'conceptual map' needs to be understood in terms of previous policy documents and earlier technologies of intervention related to child welfare. However, the Framework needs to be more expansively perceived, fixed and located as it relates to other elements in New Labour's political 'project'. It will also be argued that the Framework's preoccupation with an ecological approach to assessments and with questionnaires and scales is likely to have major implications for social work practice and for micro-engagements with children and families.

The following chapter will examine another key component of New Labour's approach to social work with children and families – the promotion of child adoption. Conservative administrations of the 1990s failed to introduce changes to the law in England and Wales, yet used adoption to attack 'political correctness'. New Labour's initial preoccupation centred on the Prime Minister's Review and the hyperbole surrounding its initiation (Performance and Innovation Unit 2000). The outcome of the review, it is argued, hints at a hankering for a return to an anachronistic conceptualisation of adoption and needs to be understood in terms of the Blair administration's more encompassing orientation to welfare services and the family. It is suggested, moreover, that the US influence is also significant (Deacon 2000).

Chapter 7 will then investigate social work's dominant approach to questions of 'race' and ethnicity. Here it will be maintained that Britain's largest ethnic minority – Irish people – have continually been excluded from the dominant discourse of anti-discriminatory, or anti-oppressive, social work theory (see O'Neale 2000). The main reason for this centres on the dominant tendency to exclusively centre on 'race' and visible difference. Conceptually this approach is founded on implicit ideas about British identity and erroneously suggests that white ethnicities are homogeneous, unified and clearly demarcated from a (new) black presence. In this chapter it will be argued that the mainstream and hegemonic discourse on 'race' needs, therefore, to take specific account of Irish people and other minority ethnicities not identifying as 'black', particularly during a period of new migration to Britain by refugees and asylum seekers who may not identify as 'black'. The Irish dimension is important in itself, but this chapter also provides an opening to address more general issues centred on 'race', ethnicity and social work with children and their families. This, it is argued, is particularly important given the contemporary trend in which DoH guidance and protocol documents are tending to downgrade the importance of anti-discriminatory practice.

Chapter 8 will argue that the future of what we perceive as social work with children and families remains uncertain, particularly given the growth of an array of 'mentors' and 'personal advisers'. Specifically, the chapter will focus on the 'new profession' of 'personal adviser' set up under the auspices of the new Connexions agency for thirteen to nineteen-year-olds. How are personal advisers likely to impact on social work with children and families? What does the new agency tell us about government perceptions of children and young people in this age bracket?

Chapter 9 will then form an overview and identify a number of the themes, which have emerged in the book. It will emphasise that child-care social workers clearly need to embrace change. However, it will also be stressed that, whilst being prepared to be constructively engaged with the 'modernisation' agenda, social workers, social work academics and others involved in social care need also to be *critical* agents in the process of change.

The aims of the book are relatively modest and it is, of course, conceded that, for some, it will fail to engage with their particular interests or specific concerns. Perhaps this is hardly surprising given all the areas, related to the topic, which could potentially be examined. There will not, for example, be any detailed examination of the emerging institutional framework of social work and the role of the new 'alphabet agencies' (see Jones 1999). Similarly, there will be no account of how the social work with children and families in the voluntary sector is in flux. Furthermore, more abstract – but still important – considerations related to, for example, the sociology of childhood will not be central (see Bell 1993; James and Prout 1996a; Prout 2000; Lee 2001). Neither will there be any detailed examination of issues solely related to residential care. However, at various times, all these areas will be referred to in the analysis. In brief, what the book hopes to do, amidst a flurry of initiatives centred on children and families, is to provide readers with the opportunity to 'take a step back' and to examine the remaking of social work with children and families.

Part I

MAJOR DEPARTURES?
Social work with children and families, 1990–1997

For eighteen years, social work, in Britain, was shaped by the political project of the right wing of the Conservative Party (see Gledhill 1989) which set out to 'sanitise social work' (Jones 1996a) and to rid it of any oppositional or 'ideological' infection. More specifically, social work's value base and awareness of factors connected with class, 'race', gender and oppression led to the charge of 'political correctness' (Hopton 1997; see also 'Cut the "ologies" and "isms", social workers told', *The Independent on Sunday*, 13 December 1992, and the editorial 'Who's racially naive?' *Community Care*, 9 September 1993). Social work was also tainted, in the eyes of right-wing politicians and ideologues, because of its association with the public sector and the post-war settlement between capital and the labour movement (Hall and Jacques 1989).

By the late 1990s and the fall of the Major administration, the language of market forces and market imperatives had infiltrated the theory and practice of social work and had especially come to characterise the formulations of its senior managerial, policy-making and educative tiers (Dominelli 1988; Edwards and Usher 1994; Dominelli and Hoogvelt 1996; Humphries 1997; Dominelli 1998). On this terrain, the 'social services supermarket' (Smale *et al.* 1993: 4) came to be eulogised even if this type of rhetoric was juxtaposed, not always happily (Singh 1997), with historically and professionally rooted notions such as 'traditional social work values' (British Association of Social Workers 1996) and 'anti-oppressive practice' (Froggett and Sapey 1997: 47–8).

Developments within Social Services Departments mirrored, moreover, similar changes across the public services. Central here was the spread of consumerism which entailed the introduction of the Citizens' Charter and a plethora of 'league tables' to measure 'performance' and what has been referred to, in a US context, as the gradual 'businessing of human services'

(Finn and Nybell 2001: 140; see also Clarke and Newman 1997; 'Major pledges public service "revolution"', *The Guardian*, 11 May 1991). In Britain, populist measures, such as charters and tables, were also frequently coupled with political attacks on those, such as social workers, working in the public sector who were the 'target' of 'reform'.

In the mid-1990s a debate was triggered on the 'refocusing' children's services (Aldgate 2002). Important here was an Audit Commission report, *Seen but not Heard*, published in 1994, and *Child Protection: Messages from Research*, published during the summer of the following year (Department of Health 1995a). The latter, by the Dartington Research Unit, which brought together findings from twenty separate studies, was to prove particularly influential. One of the key messages to emerge from this overview of research and the associated political interventions by Ministers was that social workers needed to use a 'lighter touch' when engaging in child protection activity (see 'Zealous child abuse investigators to be curbed by new rules', *The Sunday Times*, 15 January 1995; 'Social workers need to use "lighter touch"', *The Guardian*, 22 June 1995). As 'things stood', the authors of the 1995 report asserted: '[A]nyone in regular contact with children, however uncertain or untrained in abuse matters, had the power *to inflict child protection procedures on parents*' (Department of Health 1995a: 61, emphasis added). Somewhat controversially – given that it ran counter to the government's own guidelines – the report went on to argue that so-called 'chaotic families already supported by social workers might easily be approached *without the need to raise the spectre of a specific allegation*' (Department of Health 1995a: 16; see also Parton 1995).

This DoH report, apt to be referred to as the 'blue book', was trumpeted as heralding the 'biggest upheaval in child protection since the Cleveland scandal' ('Child abuse inquiries to be cut', *The Guardian*, 30 May 1995). This comment over-emphasises the significance of the publication and there was also reasonable suspicion, at the time, that the Major administration was cynically intent on reducing the cost of 'expensive' child protection investigations. None the less, the 'blue book' can be interpreted as significant for three reasons. First, it was conceded, perhaps for the first time in an 'official' report, that child abuse was socially constructed. Thus it was acknowledged that society 'continually reconstructs definitions of child maltreatment, which sanction intervention'. Moreover, the 'state remains selective in its concerns' (Department of Health 1995a: 15). Second, the report set out to shift the focus of child protection from a 'preoccupation with abuse events rather than with the processes that underlie them' (Department of Health 1995a: 20). Specifically significant in this context was the authors' aim of drawing attention to the poor outcomes for children living in families characterised as 'low on warmth and high on criticism' homes (Department of Health 1995a: 19; see also Scourfield

2000). Finally, the report in stressing how 'child protection' and 'family support' needed to be welded together, and not entirely separate forms of social work intervention, indicated a shift away from the forensic orientation to child abuse found in the so-called 'orange book' (Department of Health 1988). This movement – from 'orange' to 'blue' – was also to provide part of the foundation of the *Framework for the Assessment of Children in Need and their Families* (Department of Health, Department for Education and Employment, Home Office 2000).

More generally, for many children and their families, deepening poverty characterised the period of successive Conservative administrations (see Garrett 2002). In the late 1980s, for example, Bebbington and Miles (1989) found that 20 per cent of children becoming 'looked after' were from families in receipt of Income Support. Freeman and Lockhart's later research suggested that, in some areas, 75 per cent of children entering the 'looked after' system were from families relying on benefit (in Becker 1997: 111). In the late 1990s 'nine out of ten users of social services' were claiming benefits, with the majority on means-tested benefits 'reserved for the poorest' (Becker 1997: 88). Many of those in receipt of benefits – and *not* in receipt of benefits – were trapped in debt (Ford 1991).

Specific benefit policy changes also had an impact on the users of social services. Particularly prominent here was the scrapping of 'single payments' (Cohen and Tarpey 1988) and the introduction of the pernicious Social Fund under the Social Security Act 1986 (Stewart and Stewart 1986; Craig 1989; Bradshaw and Holmes 1989; see also 'Social Fund maintains cycle of debt', *Community Care*, 22–28 February 2001). This loans-based scheme which pits the poor against the poor is, of course, being maintained by New Labour (Pearce 2001a, b, c). On account of central government constraints, Social Services Departments' financial assistance to service users was also cut – in real terms – throughout the 1980s and 1990s. This was facilitated by the introduction of various 'classifications of needs', which were used to ration access to services and resources (see also Hillyard and Percy Smith 1988: ch. 6).

Throughout the 1990s, other policy departures related to housing, the NHS and education also had an impact. Walker and Walker (1998: 46) observed in the late 1990s that a

> significant proportion of the British population are living on incomes substantially below the average for the rest of the population and are, as such, at risk of malnutrition, hypothermia, homelessness, restricted educational opportunities, poorer health, earlier death and being the victims of crime. For example, a child born into a poor family is four times as likely as a child from a better-off family to die before the age of 20 [see also Jack 2000b].

Indeed, by the mid-1990s, Britain had one of the worst records on child poverty in the industrialised world, with nearly 20 per cent of children living in families below the poverty line. This compared unfavourably with countries such as Sweden, Norway and Finland which had rates of 5 per cent (Green 2000; see also '"Mass affluents" get richer as the poor get poorer', *The Guardian*, 2 April 2001).

Pervasive 'underclass' stereotypes and 'sink estate' imagery was also important and provided part of the cultural ambience for social work with children and families during the Major period. Particular neighbourhoods, or 'symbolic locations', were variously described as part of 'No-go Britain' (Victor *et al.* 1994; Loos 1994) and 'estates from hell' (see Campbell 1995a; Melkie 1997; Garrett 2001). Related to this, but also connected with the murder of James Bulger, there were concerns about wayward, or unruly, children (see also Valentine 1996). Emblematically, in the early 1990s, for example, a 'public awareness exercise' about the threat of car crime portrayed young men as hyenas. Meanwhile, a 'rat boy' was reported to be skulking in the detritus and ventilation shafts of tower blocks on Newcastle's Byker estate. More fundamentally, the Major period also saw the re-emergence, alongside discourses centred on children 'at risk', of a 'wide range of shadow concerns about "risky children" regarded as significant threats to society' (Stephens in Finn and Nybell 2001: 141).

Importantly, all these developments, provided, therefore, part of the political and sociological backdrop for the emergence of the Looking after Children (LAC) system. This period also saw – despite some reservations in the 'blue book' (Department of Health 1995a: 38) – the creeping criminalisation of child welfare discourses and a much closer joint working relationship between social workers and police officers in the context of child protection. The following three chapters will, therefore, examine these developments in greater detail.

2

THE 'BLUEPRINT' FOR CHANGE
The 'Looking after Children' system

'Towards a Blueprint of Parental Tasks and Responsibilities'.
(Ward 1995c: 60)

In the mid-1990s there were, in England alone, approximately 50,000 children and young people 'looked after', excluding those disabled children receiving respite care (Department of Health 1996: 5). Moreover, the case for wholesale reform of the public care system was powerful and persuasive, particularly if account was taken of local authorities' historical and contemporary shortcomings with regard to the children for whom they had responsibility (Hendrick 1994; Utting 1997). The Waterhouse inquiry on abuse in North Wales children's homes (Waterhouse 2000; see also Thompson 1998; Pritchard 1998) and a number of other inquiries focused on the harm caused to children in institutional and substitute family environments (Staffordshire County Council 1991; Westcott 1991; Lyon 1997). In addition, research highlighted: the inadequate health provision available for 'looked after' children (Butler and Payne 1997), their poor level of educational achievement (Jackson 1988–9; Heath et al. 1989; Aldgate et al. 1993; Fletcher-Campbell 1998); the bullying taking place in 'care' settings (Colton 1989) and the lack of independent visitors (Utting 1997: 111–12); the high pregnancy rates of young women 'looked after' (Corlyn and McGuire 1998); the specific problems encountered by black children and young people (Chambers 1998); the unacceptably high number of placement moves (Sone 1997a); the inadequacy of preparation for 'leaving care' and poor after-care support (Biehal et al. 1995). Clearly, there should have been profound concern about the well-being of 'looked after' children and young people, both in terms of their day-to-day experiences and their longer-term opportunities.

However, the academics associated with the *Looking after Children: Assessing Outcomes in Child Care* project, mindful of this situation, boldly asserted that their new system would contribute to the final shedding of the 'painfully persistent legacy of minimum standards and minimum objectives

19

that was inherited from the Poor Law' (Parker *et al.* 1991: 74). *Action and Assessment Records* (AARs), the centrepiece of the LAC system, were designed to assess 'looked after' children's progress from birth into young adulthood by means of a series of questions which according to the scheme's *Training Guide* would seek 'objective answers' (Department of Health 1995b: 58). These were to be used with children located in six different age bands: under one year, one to two years, three to four years, five to nine years, ten to fourteen years, fifteen years and over. Other LAC materials were – and remain – available and these form an integrated package of documentation. As well as the ARR booklets there are: *Essential Information Records* Part 1 and Part 2; a *Care Plan*; a *Placement Plan* Part 1 and Part 2; three sets of Consultation Papers and a Review of Arrangements form.

The main argument to be developed in this and the following chapter, however, is that the scheme – so central to the remaking of social work with children and families – lacks sociological curiosity and elides a constellation of key questions. None the less, until the intervention of Knight and Caveney (1998), no critique of the LAC system had appeared in the social work literature and the seemingly benign and hegemonic vision of the scheme's proponents remained unchallenged. What follows, though, is not an attempt to provide a crude, or even conspiratorial, account of the LAC scheme, because it is recognised that social policy formulation and implementation are highly complex (see Hill 1993). Rather, the aim is simply to prise open aspects of the LAC enterprise, which have been closed down and rarely interrogated. In brief, the suggestion is that the *arrival* of the LAC system needs to be situated within a wider and more embracing analytical framework than has been provided by the scheme's academic designers (for example, Parker *et al.* 1991; Ward 1995a). The aim will be to focus specifically on the potentially damaging aspects of the LAC system and to provide a critique of facets of its conceptualisation. Furthermore, the 'discrowning' of LAC (Bakhtin in Irving and Young 2002: 25) remains necessary because of the welter of uncritical contributions from the academics associated with the project and the lack of a more sceptical countervailing discourse. Indeed, the whole LAC enterprise, with its 'homogenizing expert narrative' (Leonard 2000: 164), needs to be examined in analytical and critical depth, if only because, as Knight and Caveney (1998: 31) observe: 'the history of child care in Britain is littered with solutions that subsequently emerged as creating problems themselves'.

This chapter will, therefore, focus on a number of key features of the LAC system. First, its discourse on parenting will be examined. This will be followed by an exploration of how the system relates to contemporary concerns about 'troublesome' young people (see James and Jencks 1996; Henricson 2000). In conclusion, the chapter will provide a critical and detailed examination of the AARs.

The LAC system and parenting

At the heart of the LAC system remains an extraordinary ambition, even conceit: an academic and technocratic project, according to its *Training Guide*, to identify and codify 'explicitly what good parenting means in practice' (Department of Health 1995b: 22). The aim now, therefore, is to interrogate the main features of the LAC system's perspective on parenting. This will include an exploration of focal ideas about 'corporate parents' and 'reasonable' parents and an examination of the 'community study' which underpins the LAC approach.

Corporate parents

'Parenting' is central to the LAC scheme and local authorities are repeatedly described as 'corporate parents' of the children and young people who are 'looked after' (see Jackson *et al.* 1996). As Miller (1998) asserts 'corporate parenting' is 'one of the buzz phrases in social care at the moment' and in the late 1990s it was again officially emphasised in the New Labour administration's Quality Protects (QP) initiative for local authority children services (Department of Health 1998a, b; Dobson 1998; Hirst 1998). However, the phrase and conceptualisation, first given a type of intellectual substance and then popularised within the LAC discourse, remain somewhat problematic.

Clearly, a local authority can have 'parental authority' for a child, under the Children Act 1989, although this remains a purely legal construct. To begin with, it might be argued, perhaps pedantically, that an inorganic entity – a local authority – cannot be *a parent*. More fundamentally troubling, however, the 'corporate parent' construct might be perceived as marginalising, even disparaging, a child or young person's *actual* parent(s) with whom the local authority is supposed to be working in partnership (Department of Health 1995c: 14; Jackson *et al.* 1996: 9–13). Indeed, the specificity of the actual parental relationship was acknowledged some years ago in terms of the vocabulary of social work with, for example, the redesignation of *foster parents* as *foster carers*. In this sense the concept of *corporate parent* can, perhaps, be understood as a retrograde step.[1]

Moreover, in the mid-1990s, when the LAC scheme first began to have an impact, some 39 per cent of 'looked after' children were voluntarily accommodated under section 20 of the Children Act 1989 and the local authority did not even possess 'parental responsibility' (Department of Health 1996: 5). Thus it is incorrect to state that, with *all* 'looked after' children, 'agencies which undertake the care of children separated from their family . . . *assume* parental responsibility for them' (Ward 1993: 229, emphasis added). A further 9 per cent of children on care orders were living with their actual parent(s) (Department of Health 1996: 12), yet this group (4,300 in England alone in 1995) simply did not feature in the any of the commentaries associated with the LAC scheme. Rather, it was erroneously implied that all 'looked after' children were living either in foster placements or in children's homes (see, for example, Parker *et al.* 1991; Ward 1995a) despite the fact that the number of children in community homes had been declining since the early 1980s: from 14,794 in 1985 to 9,710 in 1991, 6,400 in 1994 and 6,000 in 1995 (Department of Health 1996: 6). Similarly, with the LAC literature, there was no reference to those children and young people who were the subject of care orders, but placed with relatives assessed as foster carers. All this suggests that the academics associated with the LAC project perhaps failed to adequately delineate who exactly comprised the 'looked after' group of children and young people.

Reasonable parents

The construct of a 'reasonable parent' is found, but not defined, in section 31 of the Children Act 1989, and, in fact, the designers of the LAC scheme contend that the 'good local authority will mirror the practices of the reasonable parent' (Parker *et al.* 1991: 63). As observed earlier, in the LAC *Training Guide*, it was unequivocally asserted that the scheme 'sets out explicitly what good parental care means in practice' (Department of Health 1995b: 22). However, despite the confidence of such repeated claims, the notions of 'reasonable parent' and 'good parental care' are clearly socially constructed and shift in meaning, both historically and culturally. The not entirely dissimilar construct of 'good enough parenting' (Adcock and White 1985) can be recognised as presenting similar problems because such ambiguities are not explored. Polansky *et al.*'s (1983) discussion of 'an American standard of childcare', for example, has informed the 'good enough parenting' discourse (see Adcock and White 1985: 108–13), but this can also be viewed as founded on particular class and gender-based assumptions.

Within the literature centred on the LAC system, one of the few references to the fact that ideas pivoting on the 'reasonable parent' and similar notions might be culturally and historically fluid and unstable appears in Ward (1995c: 63–4), yet this only served to highlight the LAC proponents' lack of awareness of the material hardship faced by many families in contact with Social Services Departments. It was concluded that the definition of 'well-being' implicit in the AARs was unlikely to 'become definitive and permanent' because:

> We have defined well-being in the context of British society in the 1990s. For instance, in a society where welfare provisions are minimal and survival the overriding preoccupation, helping children to

acquire a strong sense of identity may well be regarded as a frivolous side issue compared with the need to ensure they are sufficiently healthy and acquire appropriate skills to take their place in the labour market.

What the author fails to understand is that this 'other society' *was* Britain for many children and their families in the 1990s. Indeed, by the mid-1990s, when the LAC project was evolving, Britain had one of the worst records of child poverty in the industrialised world with nearly 20 per cent of children living in families below the poverty line. According to the quarterly bulletin published by the Department for Work and Pensions, even in February 2001 – after New Labour committed itself to fighting child poverty – 2.63 million children (19 per cent of children in Britain) were living in families claiming benefits. In the London area the figure was as high as 29 per cent. Of all children living in families on benefits, 61 per cent had been on benefits for at least two years (www.dwp.gov.uk).

The *silence* within the LAC discourse on poverty mirrored, moreover, that of the Thatcher and Major administrations on the subject. In short, the LAC system, whilst professing to seek to improve 'outcomes' for children and mapping out the route to achieve that aim, appeared to be an intensely insular project to the extent that it lacked interest in one of the reasons *why* children became accommodated. More specifically, the system lacked the analytical depth and vision to focus on the issue of mass poverty and the material hardship faced by many children and their families.

Perhaps, more broadly, the LAC system's parenting discourse can, however, be situated within a wider populist and authoritarian framework. During the period of Conservative Party hegemony, for example, defining ideas about the task of parenting found expression in key social policy interventions, and ideological continuity is, it will be suggested later, clearly apparent in New Labour's approach. The LAC scheme appears to mesh with a number of these developments. Ward (1995c: 61), for example, in a discussion revealingly entitled *Towards a Blueprint of Parental Tasks and Responsibilities*, argues that 'in recent years there has been considerable concern expressed both by politicians and academics that parents are increasingly uncertain of their responsibilities'. Thus, this comment tried to fuse the LAC system with a wider, more embracing, debate. The same author continues, 'concerns about cultural relativism and the erosion of responsibility have also been expressed . . . by *serious* academics' (emphasis added). However, her reference to 'serious academics' is primarily to Dennis and Erdos (1993), whose work, published by the right-wing Institute of Economic Affairs, was criticised by a number of writers for ignoring the impact of mass poverty on families and for seeking to ideologically reinforce patriarchal relationships (see also Dennis 1993; Scraton 1997).

Parenting and the 'community study'

It was vital, given the ideological disposition of the designers of the LAC system, that they were able to argue that there existed a consensual model in relation to the 'good parental care' construct. Furthermore, if they were able to do this they would, perhaps, have gone some way to rebutting the charge that their notion of parenting was rooted in a particular view of the world, or simply in 'middle-class' perceptions. This latter concern was, moreover, acknowledged, since their research endeavours raised 'questions at an early stage in the development work about the applicability of the materials beyond the aspirations of white middle-class researchers' (Jones *et al.* 1998: 220).

In arriving at an understanding as to how the 'reasonable parent' seeks a 'good outcome' for their child, the scheme's designers relied, we are told, on 'research findings and professional judgement'. Their ideas are in part, therefore, rooted in a dominant child-care discourse and, in Foucauldian terms, in particular 'regimes of truth'. We are also advised that they rigorously endeavoured to test the validity of their ideas on parenting by means of a 'community study' with children 'growing up in their own "average" families' who were 'neither especially advantaged or disadvantaged' (Parker *et al.* 1991: 52; see also Moyers and Mason 1995). Subsequently, this 'community study' has frequently been deployed in order to provide evidence of the reliability and validity of the AAR approach to the assessment of children and young people who are 'looked after' (Ward 2000a, b). The study, we are told, discovered that '*virtually* all parents' shared the views of the researchers on the key tasks of parenting and so it was concluded that there existed a consensus on parenting which dispelled those early concerns about the impact of social class location (Ward 2000a: 547, emphasis added).

As observed, this 'community study' has been repeatedly used to try and substantiate the researchers' assertions on parenting and child development, yet, despite the research data not being published, problems are still identifiable. The word 'community' – like 'empowerment' (Margolin 1997; Forrest 2000) – is one of those sentimental and seductive words which is frequently used to cover up problematic issues which are rooted in questions of domination and structural exploitation (see Anthias and Yuval-Davis 1993). Here is not the place to explore this dimension, suffice it to note that in Britain and the United States one can also temporally connect 'community' – its associations and meanings – with the discourse of communitarianism (Etzioni 1995; Campbell 1995b; Jordan 1998, Jordan 2000: 52). With the LAC research, parents who were *not* in contact with social services, in just two local authorities, took part. This 'community study' also excluded the parents of children under the age of three, and children were 'clustered' around particular age bands (Moyers and Mason 1995: 67).

Significantly, in the light of problems later encountered in relation to the use of AARs with disabled children, this school-based study also excluded 'special schools' attended by children with a range of physical and educational 'special needs'.

Elsewhere, it also becomes apparent that many other parents and their understanding of the task of parenting were excluded. Ward (1995b: 24–5) concedes that 'in spite of being able to pay an interview fee, we found that in some of the more deprived (*sic*) districts substantially fewer families were able to participate than in other areas'. In short, the 'community study' may not have been representative of the entire 'community'. However, the LAC researchers do not appear, in the light of the absent families, to have pondered on the reliability and validity of their study: might their findings be impaired on account, for example, of the social class of the remaining respondent families? Were there any specific factors connected with 'race' and ethnicity here? No evidence is, however, provided to suggest that these potentially messy, perhaps political, issues were interrogated. Instead, the parents who opted to absent themselves from the 'community study' were portrayed as deviant.

> We can only speculate about this [the non-completion of the AARs used in the community study] although it could be argued that it was the dysfunctional families, whose children are most likely to have similarities to those who are cared for by a public agency, who were the least willing to be interviewed. If this is true, it may be that the resulting data are biased in favour of the more functional families in the community.
>
> (Ward 1995b: 25)

In a less than convincing way, therefore, many parents and perhaps their differing perceptions and approach to parenting were pushed out of the analytical frame. Methodologically, this fails to satisfactorily address a range of concerns associated with research interviews (Gudmundsdottir 1996; Kvale 1996): for example, specific issues related to power dynamics involving the interviewer and respondent, literacy problems, the location chosen to undertake the interviews, etc. In short, the research orientation of the LAC academics was not interested in the interactive aspect of research processes or, indeed, in those facets of micro-engagements which are, for some, at the heart of social work practice with children and families (Parton and O'Byrne 2000; Taylor and White 2000; Trinder 2000: 33–4).

The dismissive attitude is partly attributable to the researchers' own values and structural location. However, it can also be connected with a more encompassing and seemingly relentless rational-technical pursuit to produce orderly and tidy explanations and to erase ambiguity (Fawcett and Featherstone 1998: 70; see also Bauman 2000a, b). Coupled with this, one finds an implicit moralising tone and the tendency to attribute 'blame' (Knight and Caveney 1998). In this sense, LAC's primary definers are, perhaps, oddly similar to those bourgeois reformers in the COS, referred to earlier, who energetically endeavoured to reshape social work and improve 'outcomes' amongst the 'industrial residuum' in the late nineteenth century (Bosanquet 1895; Woodroofe 1962; Rooff 1972).

The LAC system, 'children' and 'childhood'

Clearly, problems can be identified with ideas about 'parenting' in the LAC literature. Similarly, within the materials associated with the LAC scheme there is no detailed discussion seeking to explore how conceptualisations such as 'childhood' or 'children's needs' are arrived at and how they are apt to be contested and to shift across time and space (Parker *et al.* 1991; Corrick *et al.* 1995; Department of Health 1995b; Ward 1995a; Jackson and Kilroe 1996; Ward 1996; Jackson 1998; see also Woodhead 1990; Shamgar-Handelman 1994; James and Prout 1996a). More specifically, the design of the AARs mirrors the teleological approach which characterises developmental psychology (see Archard 1993: ch. 3; Burman 1994: ch. 4; White 1998b). Perhaps this orientation is not entirely surprising, given 'the hegemony of perspectives on childhood that come from theories of individual development or pedagogy . . . which reduce the child to a "not yet person"' (Oldman 1994: 43). However, the key criticism of this dominant perspective remains pertinent; that it risks children being regarded more as 'human becomings' than as 'human beings' (Qvortrup 1994: 4).

It might, of course, be countered that issues such as this are somewhat 'abstract' and a diversion from the pragmatic, 'commonsense', professional task of 'improving outcomes' for all 'looked after' children. Indeed, the LAC system, according to its *Training Guide*, 'directs attention to concrete matters and away from more abstract considerations' (Department of Health 1995b: 60). None the less, the whole LAC enterprise can be interpreted in a more expansive way as being founded, as we shall see, on a social construction of a *particular* group of children at a *particular* moment in history. Important, in this sense, is how it can be connected with discourses fixated on *some* children as a threat to civil order.

Protecting the community from children 'in care'

Children are 'now at the centre of political strategies in late modernity' (James *et al.* 1998: 8) and specifically relevant here is the fact that the LAC scheme was, perhaps, informed by contemporary concerns (and fears) about children, and especially marginalised children, in the 'care' of local authorities. This point is pertinent because the literature centred on the system fails to situate contemporary perceptions of children, particularly of 'troublesome' children (Newburn 1996), within its limited but carefully delineated conceptual frame of reference. More broadly, as Hendrick (1994: 8) has observed, it 'is important for a proper understanding of social policy in relation to children (and adolescents) that we recognise just how much of so-called protective legislation has been concerned with their presence as *threats* rather than as suffering *victims*'.

Indeed, children, viewed as being *at risk* of offending or as threats to communities, have often also been represented as *products* of the 'care system'. In February 1993 the then Home Secretary Kenneth Clarke made this link explicit when he attacked 'persistent, nasty little juveniles'. He also went on to lambast the 'social work profession for not succeeding with children' and concluded that 'it is no good them mouthing political rhetoric, as some of them do, about why *children in their care* are so delinquent' (*The Guardian*, 22 February 1993, emphasis added). During the early 1990s there was also something of a 'moral panic' about children which touched on a constellation of interlocking concerns (Valentine 1996). In part, this was bound up with the response to the murder of James Bulger, but it was also enmeshed with other issues concerning the alleged 'loss of childhood innocence' (*The Observer*, 18 June 1995) so-called 'dismembered' or 'fatherless' families (Dennis 1993) and the growth of an alleged 'underclass' (Murray 1990; Garrett 2002).

This theme will be returned to later in the discussion when we examine how the LAC system could relate to the identification of potential young offenders. The main point to make here is that these debates and the creeping criminalisation of the discourses of child welfare inescapably formed and continue to form part of the ideological matrix and ethos of the LAC enterprise. In short, with the LAC system different discourses centred on children in public care and combating youth crime interconnect and feature as a powerful subtext. This becomes particularly clear when the AARs are subjected to detailed investigation.

Assessing children and young people in public care: Action and Assessment Records

AARs are to be used with children 'looked after' by local authorities and are designed to improve their 'outcomes' (see also Department of Health 1998a, b). In addition, these booklets are supposed to enable Social Services Departments and the Department of Health to focus on and track developments in relation to seven key dimensions of a 'looked after' child's life:

- Health.
- Education.

- Identity.
- Family and social relationships.
- Social presentation.
- Emotional and behavioural development.
- Self-care skills.

In order to briefly explore some of the issues related to the practical use of the AARs here we will mainly confine ourselves to commenting on the booklets to be used with young people aged ten to fourteen years and fifteen years and over. A number of additional points can, however, first be made which relate to the use of the AARs to be used with children and young people in all of the five (arbitrary) age bands.

The checklist format, for example, with multiple choice answers, is potentially overly directive and alienating for young people (see Francis 2002). Furthermore, it appears that during the limited piloting of the AARs some 'adolescent' service users simply 'refused to participate' in the AAR completion exercise (Parker *et al.* 1991: 124). The attitude of these young people can be related to the clinical and interrogative format, but it might also be connected with how these booklets can be interpreted as objectifying children and young people. Butler-Sloss in the report on the Cleveland inquiry (Secretary of State for Social Services 1988) famously remarked that the child at the centre of child protection investigation was 'a person and not an object of concern', yet the LAC system appears, in many respects, to invert this maxim. This was even more apparent with earlier versions of the AARs, where, for example, questions asked, even to young people as old as fifteen, were to be posed to them not directly but to their social worker, or carer, who was then expected to speak *about them* and *for them*. In this way, it appeared to be suggested, the young people were, in the words of James and Jencks (1996: 329), not 'competent articulators of their own experiences'. Even with the revised materials, dangers continue to exist in that the harsh impersonal rigour of the AAR approach could prove counterproductive to the stated aims of the designers of the documentation. That is to say, the completion of the booklets is likely to reinforce the sense of stigma and 'abnormality' a young person might already feel whilst being 'looked after' (Merrick 1996: appendix; see also Aldgate and Statham 2001: 72–3). Moreover, despite the modalities of state intervention now being entirely different, this by-product of the LAC system highlights – despite the assertions of the academics associated with the project – continuities with the Poor Law administration of child welfare.

Concerns must also exist about which section of the AARs questions are situated. Many young people are affronted by how the AAR booklet for those aged fifteen and over addresses potentially emotive and intrusive questions on alcohol, drug use and sexuality in just four pages (see also

Francis 2002: 457). Questions relating to a young person's sexual orientation are also rendered medical matters by being placed in the section headed 'Health', as opposed to 'Identity'. Similarly, working against some of the advances made by disability rights campaigners and proponents of anti-discriminatory social work practice (Forsythe 1995), the design of the AARs is founded on a medical, as opposed to social model of disability (see Oliver 1984) and a tendency exists elsewhere in the LAC literature to use discriminatory labels such as 'able-bodied' (Ward 1995b: 28). Indeed, during the piloting of the AARs, it was admitted that 'parents and carers of children with disabilities often found the whole concept difficult to accept' (Ward 1995c: 52).

Which 'race' or ethnic group do you belong to? The AARs and 'identity'

It has been conceded that it was 'difficult to obtain comments from representatives from minority ethnic groups' before the first versions of the AARs were published (Ward 1995c: 46). Why this was the case, however, has not been explained. Similarly, no explanation is available as to why neither the LAC project team nor the Department of Health established a working party or advisory group to focus solely on issues concerned with 'race' and ethnicity, despite the plethora of groups set up to address, for example, health, education and the LAC computer system (see Ward 1995a: appendix 1). Perhaps the lack of a more thorough discussion on this topic contributed to the problems which subsequently became so apparent. Certainly the vocabulary used in the sections dealing with 'race' and culture remains unsatisfactory. It was observed, for example, that 'some of the shire counties' which piloted the AARs were 'largely unaffected by immigration' (Ward 1995c: 46) and that this had an impact on the social workers completing the section on Identity. Yet this association of a black presence with 'immigration' remains starkly anachronistic and jarring.

Furthermore, a more liberal ethos, reflected in the claim that children in Britain live in a 'multi-racial society', is rendered somewhat shallow by the LAC *Essential Information Record* Part 2 which bluntly asks the social worker to note the 'immigration status if applicable', together with the child's 'Home Office registration number' (Q25): information which has little to do with ensuring that the welfare of the child is the 'paramount consideration' (Children Act 1989, section 1) and more to do with making sure that the surveillance requirements of the Home Office, historically founded on a narrow legal, even racist, construction of national identity, are met (see also Sone 1997b; Cohen 2002).[2]

It might reasonably be argued that child-care social workers should not be routinely asking the users of services their 'immigration status' and

'Home Office registration number' in the manner that this question directs them. Clearly, the issue could be pertinent in terms of the relationship with a specific family and the information might, for example, be recorded on the 'case' file. None the less, concerns remain about how this question risks undermining, or deflecting, social work engagements with some parents and their children. These families might, for example, begin to ponder the basis of social work involvement if a child is accommodated under section 20 of the Children Act 1989 after, say, child protection concerns and then this question on immigration status is subsequently posed. More fundamentally, parents who are black will perceive the question in an entirely different light from parents who are white. Indeed, Q25 cannot be viewed as a mere technical question, because it needs to be situated in the context of black people's experience of racism in Britain (see Parekh 2000).[3] The director of the African Families Foundation, for example, told the inquiry into the death of Victoria Climbié that it was difficult for members of African communities to report child protection concerns to statutory agencies on account of the legacy of colonialism (*Community Care*, 28 March–3 April 2002: 10). Indeed, if Q25 is routinely posed it might also deter some families from approaching local authority social services for services for 'children in need' because they could be wary that the local authority will routinely log their 'immigration status' and politely ask for their 'Home Office registration number' (see Sone 1997b: 21). Despite such an understanding perhaps being erroneous – and one would assume entirely at odds with the intentions of the designers of the LAC system – this factor could still impact on the behaviour of potential referrers.

Equally important, in terms of 'race' and ethnicity, the section of the AAR focusing on a 'looked after' young person's developmental progress in relation to her/his sense of Identity, promotes a static and sociologically outmoded conceptualisation of identity (Hall 1990, 1992a; Dominelli *et al.* 2001). This is partly because of the checklist format, which does not lend itself to complex, nuanced understanding. However, a static and stable construct of 'race' and ethnicity is also to blame. Thus, one of the questions for young people aged fifteen years and over asks 'Do you know what race or ethnic group you belong to?' (ID8). The completion options allow for 'Yes,' 'No,' 'Not sure.' This is then followed by 'How would you describe yourself (e.g. black, white, Italian, Asian, Chinese, African)?' Leaving aside the exclusion of the largest ethnic group in Britain – Irish people – from this list of examples (see Hickman and Walter 1997), this simplistic orientation also fails to allow for a child or young person having a sense of dual or multiple racial or ethnic identities. The approach found in the AARs encourages, therefore, fixed categorisation and compartmentalisation which might be suitable for the gathering of aggregate statistical information for computer databases but is likely to fail to satisfactorily embrace the complexity of issues experienced by young people in relation to their 'race', or ethnicity. As Knight and Caveney (1998: 36) assert, the entire LAC response to such questions reflects a certain 'naivety' of conceptualisation and appears also to be 'reducing the significance of "race" and culture in the same way as traditional psychology has done' (see also Burman 1994).

Identifying 'problem behaviours': the AARs and 'Emotional and Behavioural Development'

Furthermore, a number of the questions featured in the AAR schedules imply that value judgements are being made about an 'appropriate way to live' and 'appropriate lifestyles': for example, 'looked after' young people, aged fifteen and over are asked about their 'wedding' arrangements (F9). The section of the AARs exploring a young person's Emotional and Behavioural Development is also troubling. Ward (1993: 229) makes it plain that this particular section of the AARs 'is largely confined to the management of problem behaviours', which is 'very often the reason for a local authority's involvement with a family'. This comment, therefore, roots the assessment approach in the understanding that the behaviour of 'looked after' young people is likely to be problematic and erroneously implies that such behaviour probably prompted the initial involvement of the local authority, yet no empirical research is marshalled to substantiate this notion. More fundamentally, this idea fails to take account of those children and young people who initially began to be 'looked after' under the Children Act 1989 not because of professional concern about *their* behaviour but because of the abusive and harmful behaviour of their parents or carers. Moreover the questions young people are to be asked, in this section of the AAR, are very crude and appear to be in danger of seeking to entirely 'medicalise' children's difference, distress or defiance. Earlier versions of the AARs also included, for example, overtly authoritarian questions asking about a child or young person's 'habitual defiance at school or home'.

In the revised versions of the AARs the first part of this section is a questionnaire – consisting of thirty questions – which is based on 'the Rutter Scales and similar instruments' (Quinton 1996: 52). These questions focus on: a child or young person's relationship with others, their concentration and behaviour, their anxieties and worries. The task for both the carer and the 'looked after' young person is to complete this questionnaire since it is 'like a screening test for a physical problem' and a 'total score' can then be arrived at which 'shows the overall level of difficulties'. In addition, 'sub-scores' can also 'indicate the kind of problems the young person is experiencing' (Quinton 1996: 52). This is of concern not only because the AARs fail to make it explicit that this type of test can subsequently result in a 'score' being calculated which might later have diagnostic consequences.

It is also worrying because interventions in 'the lives of children and young people because of their "disturbed" behaviour can escalate into a spiral of increasing restriction' (Coppock 1996). More generally, perhaps we should remain mindful of the social and temporal context in which these 'tools' are used. For, as Janet Finn and Lynn Nybell (2001: 139) have asserted, 'talk of globalisation, transnationalism and a "new world order" has co-incided with a proliferation of new forms of pathology by which troubled children and troubling youth are classified and treated' (see also 'Schools forcing children to take drug, parents say', *The Observer*, 22 April 2001).

In this same section of the AAR a young person over the age of ten years is asked, 'Have you been cautioned by the police or charged with a criminal offence within the last six months?' Followed by 'If not, have you done anything that might have got you into serious trouble (e.g. theft, drug-dealing, riding in stolen cars, fire setting, vandalism) within the last six months?' (B3). Clearly, this very much relates to concern about the delinquency of young people 'in care' and to the increasing criminalisation of child welfare discourses and practices referred to earlier. More specifically, perhaps, it also reflects a preoccupation with the types of crime committed by male youth (see Campbell 1993). Girls who are 'looked after' – and in 1998 they comprised 45 per cent of children in this group – are likely to be particularly confused – or affronted – by this line of questioning (Department of Health 1998c: 4). Crassly, these questions on criminal activity are also situated immediately before a question asking whether the young person has experienced sexual abuse (B4).

The normal child in the normal society: the AARs and 'Social Presentation'

The section of the AARs called 'Social Presentation' merits particular attention. This process begins, we are advised, 'at an early age, when children are taught to say please and thank you' (Kilroe 1996: 47). Here again the normative and oppressive potential of the LAC system is further evidenced: implicit is a picture, or template, of a 'normal' child or young person who is able to function as a productive member of a 'normal', well ordered society. The question is posed 'Do you know how to *adjust your behaviour* and conversations to different situations (e.g. *at work*, college or school, with friends, *teachers or managers*, at home or with people who you don't know very well?' (P4; emphases added). The completion options provided are 'Yes,' 'Not always,' 'No.' The next question goes on to enquire 'Who will take further action?'

These inquiries, with their unquestioning bias towards adult authority figures (the teachers and managers) are rooted in normative assumptions and socially conformist imperatives, yet it is not, of course, perceived that way by the designers of the forms because the assumptions and imperatives are part of their 'commonsense' and world view. However, despite the take-it-for-grantedness of much of this, we have here a profoundly ideological view not only of children and young people, but also of the society in which they live. This is also clear in terms of how 'work' is represented as being unambiguously developmentally beneficial. Employment 'encourages self-esteem' and 'provides a clear sense of identity' (Parker *et al.* 1991: 90) and 'looked after' young people aged fifteen years and over are asked, for example, in the Education dimension of the AARs, whether or not they have 'a job', even 'a Saturday job' or 'paper round' (E11). All of which seems to suggest that the academics responsible for the design of the AARs hold a somewhat benign view of late capitalism and of the type of economic and social relationships it promotes (see 'Children work for 33p an hour', *The Guardian*, 11 February 1998).[4]

Indeed, specific 'messages' about 'work' and what constitute *appropriate* employee demeanours feature as powerful subtexts in the AARs. This also gels with a more embracing approach to social welfare which, as will be argued later in this book, can be identified with what has been called in the United States the 'new paternalism' (Mead 1997; King and Wickham-Jones 1999; Prideaux 2001). The prime example of this approach is to be found in the various federal and state Workfare programmes (Handler 2000), but also in the British derivative – the so-called 'New Deal' (Jordan 2000; Prideaux 2001, Department for Education and Employment 2001a, b). In late 1999, for example, it was reported that young people, aged between eighteen and twenty-four who have been unemployed for six months, would have to attend full-time courses which would 'assist' them in their search for work. Central here would be the teaching of 'behavioural skills such as discipline, punctuality and presentation' (see 'Unemployed youths face intensive job search interviews', *The Guardian*, 21 September 1999; see also 'Jobless forced to take lessons', *The Guardian*, 12 January 2000). The suggestion is that the influence of 'new paternalism' detectable in these and other social welfare policies also provides part of the political and cultural context of the LAC project which contains some of these same preoccupations. That is to say, this new 'politics of conduct' (Mead in Deacon and Mann 1999) and the LAC academics' ruminations, evidenced most graphically in the Social Presentation section of the AARs, reflects, to be sure, aspects of 'careism' (Lindsay 1998). However, the LAC project can also be related to more pervasive projects and technologies concerned with constructing and grooming young adults who will be adequately prepared and schooled for labour market commodification (see also Bauman 1998: ch. 4; Jameson 2000).[5]

Certainly an encompassing work ethic, associated with the apparent aim of producing *moral* citizens, recurs constantly in the AARs and is further reflected in an insistent and badgering emphasis on 'constructive' activities. It is underpinned by an implicit and explicit hankering to shape, structure and regulate a 'looked after' young person's temporal world: an attitude, perhaps, also connected with the 'principle of non-idleness' and the fear that 'wasting time' is also a 'moral offence' evidencing 'economic dishonesty' (Foucault 1977: 154). This regulatory impulse illuminates, in part, an endeavour to bring about what Ennew (1994: 127) refers to as the 'curricularisation' of the non-school activities of childhood and it has also been evidenced by the issuing of government guidance by New Labour on how much time each night children should spend doing homework (see 'Blunkett sets homework quotas', *The Guardian*, 22 April 1998; 'Night school in the living room', *The Guardian*, 23 April 1998). Social policy interventions such as these are, of course, also driven by the needs of capital in the context of market competition and globalisation (see Dominelli and Hoogvelt 1996). An additional factor, though, is the 'assumption that children left to themselves, idling with friends, will inevitably drift towards crime' (Coward 1997) – a notion which, as argued earlier, had particular resonance in relation to 'looked after' children and young people during the period of the LAC scheme's evolution.

In the Social Presentation section the social worker is also asked, in the 'Assessment of Objectives' part of the booklet, if the young person's appearance and behaviour are acceptable. Once again, tick-boxes prompt 'Acceptable to young people and adults?' 'Acceptable to young people only?' 'Acceptable to adults only?' 'Not acceptable to either?' 'Don't know?' Aside from being remarkably crude, such an approach which seeks to 'promote the "proper" by sharpening the sights on the improper' (Bauman 2000c: 206) is, of course, highly subjective. Within the discourse centred on the LAC system, this same subjective orientation is, moreover, reflected in Kilroe's (1996: 49) comments about how being 'physically attractive' can confer advantages on children both in terms of impressing teachers and enhancing one's opportunities on the labour market. Remarks such as these, and similar comments about 'unlikeable personal habits or inappropriate behaviour' might also especially concern disabled young people and their families. More fundamentally, given this approach adopted in the LAC system, perhaps, as Lorenz (2000: 2) argues, social workers and social work academics need to reflect on the 'social work mandate' and to ask whether they should seek to foster 'the life styles and behaviours which are the responsibility' of young people themselves and 'hence expressions of their self-chosen identities'? Alternatively, should social work merely seek to 'promote and enforce those identities which conform to given conventions and structures . . . which do not allow for diversity'? Indeed, the larger conceptual framework of the entire LAC endeavour appears, in fact, to be characterised by an implicit endeavour to produce children who will *fit* when they become adults (see also Prout and James 1990; Shamgar-Handelman 1994).

The LAC system and its potential to assist in the profiling of potentially 'troublesome' children

In early 1998 it was reported that the government was planning, by 2001, to set up a national computer record on which would be logged the educational achievement of every child in Britain. Every child was, it was reported, to be given a thirteen-digit identity number, as part of this process and their progress would be tracked from the start of primary school through to university. The child's record, held on a central database controlled by the Department of Education and Employment, would also record additional information such as a behaviour record, eligibility for free school meals and the child's first language. The general secretary of the National Association of Headteachers, however, expressed concern about the civil liberties aspect of the plan and pondered about the potential for 'misuse'. Moreover, a senior official in the office of the Data Protection Registrar dubbed the mooted scheme a potential 'nightmare' given how such a system could be abused (see 'Nightmare scheme to track every pupil', *The Guardian*, 1 January 1998).

Strikingly, no similar concerns have been expressed about the LAC materials despite the scope they provide for similar 'abuse' in the form of screening and profiling a specific group of children and young people. *The Essential Information Record* Part 2 provides for a 'child identifier number' and a completed AAR contains a vast amount of information about a 'looked after' young person which ranges from – at random – how often they played with sand or ate pasta as a child to what drugs they might have gone on to use; to whether they have been sexually abused, wet the bed or rode in a stolen car. Corrick *et al.* (1995: 33) concede that there could be 'some anxieties' about the 'use which might be made of aggregate data', but the authors associated with the LAC project have not alleviated such concerns. Bullock (1995: 101) has also observed that there could be underlying fears that information produced by the AARs might be used to 'identify potential delinquents among six-year-olds, to judge parents' competence before their child is born or to produce crude league tables showing the quality of services in different local authorities'.

Such concerns are not, however, the product of unfounded anxieties in that, since the 1990s we *have*, of course, witnessed the publication of these 'crude league tables' with data for the exercise gathered from a variety of sources held by Social Services Departments. Furthermore, specifically in relation to the surveillance and profiling of the 'potentially delinquent', it needs to be recalled that other contemporary developments also provide a context for these concerns. In 1991, for example, that the Home Office was planning a scheme to identify criminals from the age of six and here teachers and other welfare agencies were envisaged as playing a key surveillance role in identifying these potential criminals. As part of this initiative, it was reported, certain 'at risk' (of offending) categories were being formulated by Ministers and their advisers ('Ministers to target six-year-olds in bid to fight lawlessness', *The Sunday Times*, 15 September 1991). Similar ideas underpinned the intervention of a spokesman for the Association of Chief Police Officers (ACPO) when, in March 1998, he suggested that future criminals could be identified at ages as young as seven or eight. Furthermore, he continued, 'such children could be identified by teachers, social workers and police acting together in the same way as is done with children at risk of abuse' ('Criminals identifiable at age 8', *The Guardian*, 4 March 1998). This approach also underpins the Crime and Disorder Act 1998 in that the Child Safety Order is specifically concerned with children 'at risk of offending' (Home Office 1998: 8). The setting up of Youth Offending Teams and the use of the 'ASSET Young Offender Assessment Profile' schedule has also led to the type of inter-agency working and sharing of information called for by the ACPO spokesman ('Why ASSET must be a real asset for YOTs', *Youth Justice News* 8, June 2001: 3; see also Home Office 1998: 7–9).

In this context, the potential of the LAC system to be used as a mechanism to facilitate the screening and profiling of 'looked after' children and young people, particularly when used in conjunction with the range of other similar materials, remains concerning. In maintaining that this furnishes yet another reason why the scheme needs to be approached with a certain reflexive caution, one is not, however, seeking to conjure up an Orwellian or dystopian nightmare. Indeed, it is now 'hard to find a place, or an activity, that is shielded or secure from some purposeful tracking, tagging, listening, watching, recording of verification devise' (Lyon 2001a: 1). We now live, in short, in a 'surveillance society' (Lyon 2001a). However, within this society, children are 'arguably more hemmed in by surveillance and social regulation than ever before' and *particular* children are, it would appear, more subject to these processes than others (James *et al.* 1998: 7; see also 'Girl, 12, becomes youngest Briton to be tagged', *The Guardian*, 20 May 2002). This, moreover, is a theme which will be returned to in Chapters 8 and 9.

Conclusion

'Tools for practice' such as the LAC materials were formulated in a context which was – and remains – dominated by two superordinate narratives. The first is centred on the need to ensure that young people are adequately prepared for the 'world of work' and that they are compliant, well presented employees who are able to function in 'flexible' markets where national economies are compelled to compete in a global framework. The second is centred on the need to ensure that the 'crimo-genic' proclivities of the children of the unemployed and working poor are detected, regulated and contained. Put more graphically, we also need to view the remaking of social work with children and families from the direction of the 'de-regulated' workplace – where sixteen to seventeen-year olds are not afforded minimum wage protection – and the 'secure training centre'. These factors are not, to be sure, explicit in the LAC 'blueprint' for change. None the less, the interpretation provided in this chapter suggests that these are discursive components of the system which need to be analysed. This is also important because, as we shall see in the next chapter, the LAC approach continues to play such a significant role, albeit with significant refinements, in other paradigms which have been subsequently designed and implemented.

3

EXAMINING THE 'PRODUCT CHAMPIONS'

LAC and its continuing role in the remaking of social work with children and families

In many ways it remains difficult to criticise so ostensibly benign an endeavour as the LAC system. Perhaps any critic of the system also risks being unfairly positioned as wishing to maintain 'the painfully persistent legacy of minimum standards and minimum objectives that were inherited from the Poor Law' (Parker *et al.* 1991: 74). Added to this, of course, some of the LAC academics possess a good deal of 'symbolic capital' on account of their prestige and reputation (Bourdieu 1991: 231; see also Houston 2002). Furthermore, because of the association with the Department of Health, the LAC materials – in terms of their cost, style, presentation, *look* and *feel* – are loaded with weighty and authoritative connotative meanings (see Rojek and Collins 1987: 207–8; Fairclough 1999). Possibly on account of these factors, those who have published criticisms of this influential project still remain a small minority (Knight and Caveney 1998). It is, however, not without significance that 'looked after' children and young people are beginning to challenge aspects of the LAC system and are having their critical voices heard in research which examines the wider experience of being 'looked after' (see, for example, Munro 2001).

This chapter will begin by reviewing the LAC experience and examining its impact on the theory and practice of social work with children and families. It will then be maintained that it is important to analyse the LAC producers' repeated assertions that their 'product' is grounded in scholarly 'objectivity'. This notion is interrogated and then we will move on to look at the role played by the Department of Health. Specifically, it will be revealed how the LAC materials were, in fact, subject to explicit political manipulation. It is also argued that a central problem with the LAC system was its failure to incorporate children's *own* perceptions into the scheme. Examining the practical consequences for social work with children and families, we will also suggest that the introduction of the LAC system heralded a process which has seen a proliferation of centrally devised assessment schedules and other 'tools' for use with children and families.

In conclusion, it is maintained that since the early days of LAC we have also witnessed a more pervasive political preoccupation with 'outcomes' in relation to social work with children and families.

Importantly, the LAC system has, in part, failed to meet all the expectations of its academic designers. In this sense, remarks about the essentially muddled nature of policy making and prosaic factors such as 'cost constraints' and 'interdepartmental rivalries' need to be recalled (but not overemphasised) (Lewis 1986: 34; see also Newman 2001: ch. 2). Linked with this, the implementation of the system and social workers' use of the various forms have, in truth, remained somewhat 'patchy' (Bell 1998/9: 16).[1] Many social workers have also worked hard to subvert the harsh and impersonal format of AARs in order to work creatively with young people and their families. This understanding reflects, moreover, the – more general – findings of May and Buck (1998), who found, in their empirical work, that social workers still feel confident that they are able to 'salvage some spheres of discretion from "old" ways of working, whilst inventing some tactics to circumvent current restrictions' (see also Clarke and Newman 1997).

Despite these factors, the LAC system – and, just as significantly, the approach it was seeking to promote – has also met with a good deal of success and, in this sense, it continues to play a prominent role in the remaking of social work with children and families. There is, however, a need to maintain a degree of scepticism about the success of the system on account of the hyperbole generated by the schemes' creators. However, according to the LAC official *Training Guide*, by the mid-1990s 'adapted versions' of the LAC documentation were 'already being used in the United States, Canada, Australia, Norway, Belgium, Israel, the Ukraine and many other countries' (Department of Health 1995b: 20). More locally, the ubiquitous 'seven dimensions', at the heart of AARs, provide, as we shall see in Chapter 5, part of the conceptual foundation for the *Framework for the Assessment of Children in Need and their Families* (Department of Health, Department for Education and Employment, Home Office 2000). The LAC system has also influenced the emerging Integrated Children's System (ICS) which the Department of Health is hoping to implement on a national basis in 2004/5.

A continued wariness about the LAC system is important because of its, more general, uncritical acceptance in recent textbooks for social work with children and families. Brandon *et al.* (1998: 39) simply inform their readers that the LAC materials are 'likely to be useful in a range of assessment situations' and will 'better inform the worker's face-to-face work with the child'. Hayden *et al.* (1999: 50) merely note that much of 'Quality Protects can be seen as a transferral of the "Looking after Children" approach from individualistic, child-focused level of monitoring on to the broader canvas of local authority and public policy'. In short, despite the

LAC system's failure, for many social workers, to achieve 'practice validity' (in this context see Sheppard 1998), the AAR approach remains a reigning paradigm because of the way it is positioned in government, academic and Social Services Department managerial discourses (Kuhn 1966; Hughes and Sharrock 1997).

As observed, few published criticisms of the LAC system have emerged and the academic discourse on the issue has tended to be dominated by those whom Jones *et al.* (1998: 217) refer to as LAC 'product champions'. In reviewing the impact of the LAC system, it is, however, important to be open and transparent in relation to my own position, or standpoint. Saying something in relation to my subjective orientation is particularly relevant when attempting to criticise a system and a matrix of ideas which are presented as 'objective'. When I first encountered the LAC system I was a field social worker, with a full 'case load', working in a busy inner-city office. Yet, for me, it was striking that the views and perceptions of social workers were not being reflected in the academic and managerial discourse which pivoted on LAC and the use of AARs. Indeed, it appeared that any trace of social work(er) criticism, internally dialogised in the LAC discourse (particularly Ward 1995a), was rendered redundant because it was 'ideological' and at odds with the LAC promoters' 'objectivity'. More fundamentally, my sense of intellectual irritation at the 'spin' associated with the scheme was fuelled by my perception of social work's ambiguous role. That is to say, historically social work can be understood to have 'teetered between emphases on the correction of internal landscapes of individuals and families, and the insistence on correcting social environments in which individuals are located' (Rossiter 2000: 29). Since the early 1980s and 1990s, with the hegemony of the 'market society' (Taylor 1999: ch. 2), it is the former type of intervention which has become increasingly dominant. However, within the buoyant, but constrained, discourse on LAC substantial issues, rooted in social work's regulatory and disciplinary function, were masked or rendered marginal and inappropriate areas for debate. Nonetheless, in examining the remaking of social work with children and families, it remains vital to scrutinise aspects of the discourse pivoting on LAC, and central here remains the project's vaunted 'objectivity'.

The tyranny of the 'objective' account: the LAC system and the disqualification of criticism

Throughout the various reports associated with the project, such as the LAC *Reader* (Jackson and Kilroe 1996), one finds repeated and bold assertions that what we are presented with is 'objective' research. As we have seen, the LAC *Training Guide*, for example, explains that AARs feature 'a series of questions which seek *objective* answers' (Department of Health 1995b: 58, emphasis added). Elsewhere, the *Guide* maintains, without any reflexive hesitancy, or 'self-confrontation' (Beck 1994: 5), on the part of its academic authors that the LAC scheme lays out 'explicitly what good parenting means in practice'. Related to this is the tactic of positioning as 'ideological' (Jones *et al.* 1998: 217), or 'politically correct' (Ward 1995a) any comment, or perception, that runs counter to conceptualisations rooted in this professed 'objectivity'. In this way, those associated with the LAC system have tried to 'enclave as non-political matter' their own views and perceptions, and the perspectives of critical social work practitioners are rendered 'low-status' or even 'subjugated knowledge' which is persistently silenced, excluded and derided (Fraser 1989: 164; see also Humphries 1997: para. 4.6). Even the measured critique of Knight and Caveney (1998) is loftily dismissed as 'fundamentally misconceived' and 'driven more by ideological than evidential considerations' (Jackson 1998: 46). Elsewhere, Ward (1995c: 46) has argued that:

> Social workers act as advocates for the disadvantaged and it is inevitable that in the present climate, they should be enmeshed in the debate about political correctness. [However] . . . as researchers we need to retain a degree of objectivity in the face of considerable pressure.

Despite this feigned 'objectivity' and dismissal of criticism, a number of issues still need to be explored and it is unhelpful that an attempt should be made to foreclose discussion in this way.

Clearly, the LAC 'objectivist illusion' (Habermas 1996) is not sustainable and – as we saw in the previous chapter – one is able to locate the researchers' own values, own normative judgements. However, the 'ideological' taint is repeatedly used in order to disqualify practitioner criticism (Ward 1995a). In short, social workers and other critics are left grubbing around in a barren or contaminated 'ideological' domain, whilst the academics associated with the scheme – better able, of course, to avail themselves of the means to distribute their 'knowledge' – are left to occupy a pristine 'objective' sphere. They are merely reporting, in effect, on 'the way things are'. One does not have to be an epistemological or ethical relativist to suggest that, early in the twenty-first century, it is striking to find a project so confident that it has a monopoly of 'truth' (Giddens 1978; Blaikie 1993; Delanty 1997; Martinez-Brawley and Mendez-Bonito Zorito 1998; Fawcett *et al.* 2000).

Moreover, the strident tactics adopted to rebut criticism suggest the kind of 'anti-intellectualism' identified by Jones (1996b) and they also reflect a wariness and impatience with critical inquiry which might run counter to, or destabilise, dominant explanations and definitions (see also Webb 1996). Furthermore, they hint at a hankering for 'certainty' – a seeking to 'define out' the notions of 'ambiguity, complexity and uncertainty' which are, for some, at the 'core of social work' (Parton 1998: 23). Perhaps, more pro-saically, the LAC academics' response to criticism can also simply be inter-preted as merely mirroring the dominant 'can do' culture of managerialism in which it is so embedded (see also Clarke and Newman 1997).

The practical task of child-care social work is, in part, underpinned by willingness to form judgements about standards of parenting and these must be informed by reflective and considered assessments. In short, social work cannot and should not be held fast, or paralysed, by arid relativism (see Channer and Parton 1990; Parton 1990; Peile and McCourt 1997). None the less, the argument here is that we need to remain alert to how a seemingly omniscient, 'objective' discourse, such as the highly influential one which pivots on the LAC scheme, can be used to regulate and disci-pline the socially and economically marginalised children and families who make up most of the service user population. Moreover, we can continue to view the LAC system as a 'tool' which is central to the remaking of social work in terms of how it seeks to structure and steer social workers' encounters with users of social services and associated social care workers.

The alliance with the powerful: the proximity of political forces determining the content of the LAC materials

The entire LAC endeavour can, perhaps, be viewed as an energetic 'top-down' project driven by a core team of academics and senior officials in the Department of Health. In this context, a key question which remains unanswered concerns how the AARs, initially designed as 'research instru-ments', actually became 'tools' for practice? This issue is important because, in many respects, it might be suggested that the AARs retain the *look* of research questionnaires. All we are told is that the original working party established by the Department of Health was 'advised' to alter its focus, by the then ruling Conservative administration, in 1992: some five years *after* the project had been established (Ward 1995c: 38). Moreover, some evidence, which is now available, suggests that senior DoH civil servants – themselves steered by the political priorities of the Major admin-istration – maintained fairly rigid control throughout the period of the LAC system's evolution and inflation. These officials were, for example, apt to veto the publication of any research or commentary which was at odds with the aims of their political masters. Indeed, in an unsolicited letter to the author from one of the prominent social work academics asso-ciated with the LAC scheme it was commented:

> Its [the LAC system's] weaknesses partly reflect the fact that *it was developed under a Conservative government and controlled by intimi-dated civil servants that exercised tight control over the content.* The publication of the Reader [Jackson and Kilroe 1996] was delayed

for a year before we could reach any agreement with the Department of Health, which *resisted any mention of research which did not coincide with their current line as well as demanding substantial cuts*, from which the section on parenting suffered. [Emphases added.]

No doubt, as Little (1998: 5) has argued, the Department of Health 'is a house of many mansions' without a 'single view on children' services . . . there are competing perspectives'. However, at the risk of appearing crudely reductionist, this account of the constraints, which gripped the academics involved in LAC perhaps illuminates the aptness of part of Marx's famous comments on the role of ideology:

> The ideas of the ruling class are in every epoch the ruling ideas: i.e. the class which is the ruling *material* force of society is at the same time its ruling *intellectual* force. The class which has the means of material production at its disposal consequently also controls the means of mental production . . . [The ruling class] among other things rule as thinkers, as producers of ideas, and regulate the production and distribution of the ideas of their age.
>
> (Marx and Engels in Easthope and McGowan 1998)

One does not have to be a dialectical materialist or to accept Marx and Engels's entire 'grand narrative' to grasp the resonance of these observations in the current context. Despite their repeated assertions about scholarly 'objectivity', none of this is to seek to impugn the intellectual or moral integrity of the academics associated with LAC or to highlight their performative contradictions. Indeed, the content of the AARs and the plethora of associated publications are grounded in *their* 'commonsense' world view, *their* own ideological disposition. In short, the LAC system is not the product of a conspiracy because that is not how the state and government technologies function. As Rose and Miller (1992: 175) have argued:

> Central to the possibility of modern forms of government . . . are the associations formed between entities constituted as 'political' and the projects, plans and practices of those authorities – economic, legal, spiritual, medical, technical – who endeavour to administer the lives of others in the light of conceptions of what is good, healthy, virtuous, efficient or profitable. [See also Harris 1999.]

As we saw in the governmentality literature, referred to in Chapter 1, liberal government 'identifies a domain outside of "politics" and seeks to manage it without destroying its existence and its autonomy' (Rose and Miller 1992: 180). However, and as we can observe with the LAC system, 'political forces' *do* seek to 'utilise, instrumentalise and mobilise techniques and agents other than those of "the State" in order to "govern at a distance"' (Rose and Miller 1992: 181).

On account of the way the LAC project evolved, it remains critically important, therefore, that the precise degree of 'distance' from the Department of Health (and other key funders) must be a focal point of social work research agendas in the future (see also Broad 1999a). More specifically, there should be transparency and willingness not always to be aligned with dominant 'political forces', but to work creatively at the 'edge of the frame' (Martinez-Brawley and Mendez-Bonito Zorito 1998).

The failure to construct an alliance with those lacking political power: the marginalisation of 'looked after' children

Many of the problems with the LAC system stem from the fact that the researchers concerned were, perhaps, far too willing to enter into an alliance with these dominant political forces. As a result there was a failure to adequately engage with children and their families (see also Francis 2002: 450). Would, for example, the rebarbative Social Presentation section of the AARs, discussed earlier, have appeared in the form it did had this occurred? Much of this relates to the call for the 'demonopolisation of expertise' (Beck 1994: 29) and it suggests that social work academics need to form new alliances and to create new ways of working with and listening to children and young people. In this sense, the Quality Protects programme is prompting some worthwhile activity (see also, however, Munro 2001: 136).

More broadly, ideas in relation to children's rights are important in this context (Franklin 1995). Utting (1997: 109) concluded that mention of 'children's rights provokes a sour response in some quarters' and, despite rhetorically seeking the 'best outcomes' for children, the LAC research project was manifestly discomforted by the whole notion. Ward (1995c: 41–2) acknowledged the need for an 'ethical debate about children's rights', but the academics associated with LAC 'constantly found that the need for an open debate over this . . . was obscured by ideological pressures'. We are, however, magisterially advised that 'Children's wishes do not always coincide with their best interests and at times it seemed as though parents and carers were promoting their need for self-determination in order to hide their own lack of authority'. Similarly, more recently in the literature associated with the emerging Integrated Children's System (ICS), it has been confided that while 'children's recorded opinions are important in their own right, they tend to be unreliable sources of data' (Department of Health 2001c: 5). Comments such as these seek to marginalise a child's *own* perspective on social work assessments. At the same time they effectively undermine the claim that the AARs and related materials simply reflect the type of parenting provided to children by 'reasonable parents', since ultimately, it would seem, it is the academic designers who are to be the arbiters who will provide the definitive and *expert* judgements.

Little information has been published on the perceptions of 'looked after' young people themselves about the LAC scheme (see Baldry and Kemmis 1998; Munro 2001; Francis 2002). Some research has, however, highlighted how the LAC forms are 'seen as boring homework assignments that had little relevance to young people's concerns' (Aldgate and Statham 2001: 89). Four young people, who are either 'looked after' or used to be, provided contributions for a Central Council for Teaching and Training in Social Work (CCETSW) (1997: 6–11) report on students and their use of the various LAC materials. These brief contributions, largely supportive of the LAC scheme, are interesting in that they highlight the more general hardships experienced by the young people. Moreover, their comments reveal something about the indifference they have faced within the 'looked after' system, where their views were rarely sought about key aspects of their day-to-day care and the future direction of their lives. What these contributions fail to specifically reveal, however, is how the introduction of the LAC system can promote qualitative improvements. Indeed, a number of the concerns of the young people, such as those about 'subjective' opinions (CCETSW 1997: 8) being translated into facts, even labels, and social workers speaking a 'different language' (CCETSW 1997: 10) risk being magnified by the use of the AARs (see also Broad 1999b; Lewis and Lindsay 2000; Munro 2001).

More fundamentally, particular facets of the AARs can be interpreted as reflecting the LAC academics' structural and organisational separation from 'looked after' children and their families and from field social workers. These assessment 'tools' are likely to have evolved in a very different way if the researchers had, for example, engaged with ethnic minority groups in order to arrive at a more complex understanding of issues connected to 'race' and ethnicity. Would the problems associated with the AAR section on Identity have been addressed differently? The LAC academics might also have engaged with disabled children and their families (and not excluded so many from the 'community study') and disability rights campaigners. Would the medical model of disability have remained so central in the AARs had that happened? This would seem to be particularly important given that about a quarter of 'looked after' children have disabilities (Department of Health 2000a: 66).

Social workers might also have been responded to in a more constructive way had the LAC academics not been so intent on viewing practitioner contributions as 'ideology' and 'political correctness'. Would the interrogative checklist format of the AARs, so alien to the *process* of social work, have been retained? Would the hapless social worker still be required to fulfil, in effect, the role of research assistant? Perhaps, in this context, it is important to briefly review how the format of the LAC materials continues to impact on social work with children and families.

Social work's expanding 'toolbox': the impact of AARs on the *process* of social work

The 'official' promotional literature on the LAC scheme stated that the AARs are 'designed to set an agenda for meaningful conversation' (Corrick *et al.* 1995: 26). However, what the introduction of these booklets perhaps represented was the eradication of the vestigial idea that the micro-dimension of engagement and interaction with children and young people should be non-directive and empathic (see Rogers 1980). Put more theoretically, the LAC approach can also be interpreted as reflecting what Bakhtin terms 'monologism' (see Irving and Young 2002: 22). Despite the creation, for example, of so-called 'consultation forms', children's subjective experiences and rights to identify relevant issues for themselves are marginalised in the LAC approach.

Each of the AARs, discussed in the previous chapter, is devised as a checklist containing questions and an accompanying menu of multiple-choice answers with the relevant booklet for use with young people aged fifteen and over, for example, spanning sixty pages and containing approximately 375 questions. This format cannot, of course, lend itself to ease of dialogue between a social worker, or carer, and a young person because it is structured in such a directive and interrogative way. Indeed, this format mirrors but deepens and extends the approach of the now widely discredited 'orange book' risk assessment schedule (Department of Health 1988) and also reflects the competence-driven checklist approach which characterises the attainment of social work accreditation (CCETSW 1995).

As observed, an unresolved tension also exists with the AARs and this is related to the fact that they were not initially even designed as 'tools' of social work practice, but were constructed, by academic researchers, as 'research instruments'. Indeed, despite the widespread use of the forms they still bear the hallmarks of the purpose for which they were designed and intended. This is most apparent in terms of how a completed AAR, with its crude and alienating lettering and numbering system, so readily lends itself to inputting on a computer database (see, in this context, Poster 1990: ch. 3). This approach also lends itself, therefore, to fixed categorisation and compartmentalisation which might be appropriate to the gathering of aggregate statistical information but it is unlikely to satisfactorily embrace the complexity of issues centred on a young person's social and psychological development (see also Francis 2002: 458).

A further consequence of the introduction of the LAC system (and other 'tools' subsequently introduced which have built on it) is that the social worker risks becoming a mere collator of 'data'. Of course, it might be countered that the AARs are not to be used mechanistically with children and young people. Notwithstanding such an assertion, the form in which the AARs are presented is clearly likely to structure the process of engagement. Today this fundamental ambiguity in relation to the design of the AARs is, moreover, slowly beginning to be acknowledged by the Department of Health, even though it is unclear how this might begin to impact on the design of subsequent materials. It has been noted, for example, that:

> There appears to be considerable confusion over the purpose of AARs: are they data collecting instruments for use of practitioners and managers or are they personal and private documents for service users? One reason why implementation may appear to be so poor is that in authorities where the latter view is taken, the AARs are often kept separate from files and are sometimes held personally by the young people concerned – in these circumstances they are not accessible to researchers or auditors.
>
> (Department of Health 2001c)

Mindful, therefore, that the AARs were – and for some remain – 'research instruments', complex ethical problems must continue to arise concerning whether 'looked after' children and young people are, in fact, simply being used as 'research objects'. In their discussion of research ethics Roberts and Welland (1997) assert that children in 'institutional care have been particularly prone to well-meaning experimentation'. Indeed, this must be the case, not only because of power imbalances, but because the children and young people are, in a sense, a potentially *captive* researched population (see also Mauther 1997).

The impact of the LAC project on the *work* in social work with children and families remains significant, in that the use of the various questionnaire schedules, particularly the AARs, can be viewed as promoting a closely regulated 'curriculum' and also deepening the process of social work's incremental deskilling, deprofessionalisation and fragmentation. Uncritical use of the LAC materials with DipSW candidates must also prompt concern about how students are taught to perceive social work (Ward 2000a). The arid format of the AARs, for example, implicitly defines social work with children and families and conveys powerful messages about its key tasks and functions, rendering a complex world flat and uncomplicated.

The social work process promoted by the LAC system provides evidence of a reinvigorated form of Taylorism, with complex tasks being broken down into discrete components. This, moreover, facilitates social work being undertaken by less qualified staff, such as 'family support workers', or sessional and agency staff receiving lower rates of pay (Dominelli and Hoogvelt 1996; Watson 2002). Perhaps, also, the LAC enterprise encompasses and reflects more far-reaching changes in the status of 'expertise' (Rose 1993). In this context, Smith (1997: 3), for example, has pointed to the 'growing concentration on the externally measurable element of practice (performativity) rather than the internal, and relatively intangible, quality of relationships (caring)'. In this situation, the task of caring risks becoming entirely formalised, dispassionate and merely functional. Indeed, drawing on Foucault (1977: 184–94) again, the ideas and procedural orientation at the centre of the LAC endeavour, particularly the AARs, can be interpreted as, perhaps, reflecting aspects of the 'examination . . . surrounded by all its documentary techniques' making 'each individual a "case"' and fixing each subject in her or his 'own particularity'. Certainly, these techniques of judging, measuring and comparing with others aptly characterise the AAR approach. The same techniques can, moreover, now be seen to operate at an organisational level and across authorities, and central in this process is the notion of 'outcomes'.

'What works' and 'outcomes'

Part of the appeal of the whole 'outcomes' approach lies in its 'common-sense' and implicit impatience with the ambiguities and uncertainties which characterise social work (Parton 1998; Taylor and White 2000; Munro 2001). Ideas about 'outcomes' were also at the core of LAC from the outset (see also Fuller and Petch 1995: 4; Beresford and Evans 1999: 672; Parton 1999). As a senior consultant associated with the LAC scheme stated, the implementation of the system should not be seen by local authorities as 'a one-off project but as a continuous project at the heart of children's services'. Moreover, there 'was a need to establish a "measurement" culture within which the measuring of input, processes, outputs and outcomes was embodied'. This information would also be used to 'compare performance across authorities, teams and units'. Importantly, also, this rigorous promotion and managerial enforcement of the 'outcomes' and 'measurement' culture was closely bound up with the 'targeting' of resources and with using 'finite resources in the best possible way'.[2] Furthermore, during the Major period, it was clear that even if 'measurement' highlighted a shortfall or deficit in the resourcing of, for example, the child-care plans for 'looked after' children and young people, it would not result in more resources being made available, since aggregate data would, according to the system's *Management and Implementation Guide*, simply help departments 'to target resources appropriately' (Corrick *et al.* 1995: 33).

The outcomes perspective and related ideas, moreover, were not only central to the social welfare agenda of the Conservative Party, they also remain integral to the vision of the New Labour administration (see Pinnock and Garnett 2002). This was evidenced, for example, by the then Scottish Health Minister, Sam Galbraith, when he told the British Association of Social Workers (BASW) that social workers were 'too involved in processes' and insufficiently concerned with 'results' (see Mitchell 1997). Farther afield, in the United States, the Clinton administration endeavoured to change the child welfare policies of the Department of Health and Human Services to make agencies more 'outcome orientated' (Maza 2000; US Department of Health and Human Services, Administration for Children and Families 2000). Driven by concern about the escalating 'costs' of welfare, it is not without significance that the initial outcomes discourse centred on the 'corrections' sector in the United States and the alleged failure of penal and probation services to adequately contain and regulate the 'dangerous classes' and 'criminal' populations (Shaw and Shaw 1997; see also Nellis 1999: 301). In the United Kingdom this results-orientated approach to intervention and the related preoccupation with 'evidence-based' practice first found favour in health and probation services (Atherton 1999; Macdonald 1999; see also Webb 2001; Harrison 2002; Sanderson 2002). However, in social work the approach is increasingly dominant and is stressed, of course, in QP, the Framework and in the setting up of the SCIE (Department of Health, Department for Education and Employment, Home Office 2000; Department of Health 2001d; see also Jordan 2000: 206–9).[3] A publication from ADSS, heavily influenced by developments in the United States, particularly in the states of Vermont and Missouri, has also called for a more outcomes-based approach to child-care services in Britain (ADSS 2002a).

These developments can be viewed as reflecting a more pervasive concern about the way health and welfare systems must be 'seen to work', promote social order and not act as a brake on the process of capital accumulation. Furthermore, the 'outcomes' orientation inescapably connects with the operation of 'quasi-markets' in welfare services (Williams and Webb 1992; see also Clarke and Newman 1997). When compared with developments in adult services, it appears that local authorities have been reluctant to 'contract out' children's residential care (see Holden 2002). However, during the 1990s there was a marked increase in the scale of independent-sector provision in this area. In England, during the period 1993/4 to 1996/7, local authorities' own provision of residential care for children fell from 63 per cent to 53 per cent of the total (in Kirkpatrick *et al.* 2001: 53). Evidence suggests, moreover, that this has led to more children being moved out of their locality. More generally, the 'market has been problematic, both in economic and policy terms' (Kirkpatrick *et al.* 2001: 65; see also Clark 2002). However, this market in children's services can be related to the LAC approach in so far as crude 'outcome' data – available from LAC and innumerable other sources – contributes in the process of drawing up contractual specifications (see also, in this context, Youth Justice Board 2002a).

Conclusion

An examination of the continuing impact of the LAC system will be returned to in Chapter 5 when we look at the ways in which *the Framework for the Assessment of Children in Need and their Families* is, in part, built on the LAC approach to assessment. Thus far this exploration of the remaking of social work with children and families has concentrated on sources 'from above' and so we have largely been preoccupied with a close reading of the LAC materials. Nonetheless, it is also important to scrutinise what is happening 'on the ground'. More specifically, there is a need to listen to what social workers and associated staff have to say about the nature of their tasks and functions during a period of great change. The next chapter, therefore, will shift the focus to examine an aspect of the 'working together' paradigm which is at the core of 'child protection'.

4

'WORKING TOGETHER' TO PROTECT CHILDREN?

The notion of 'working together' has been central to the remaking of social work with children and families since the mid-1980s and it is, therefore, important to explore this dimension. Furthermore, in the early twenty-first century the inquiry into the death of Victoria Climbié, once again, placed the spotlight on the alleged failure of all child welfare organisations to adequately co-operate to safeguard and protect vulnerable children (Department of Health 2001b). In the Climbié case, social workers in the London Borough of Haringey, for example, were reported to have simply 'stopped attending crucial information-sharing meetings because they felt ignored by their health colleagues' (see the editorial 'There must be respect', *Community Care*, 15–21 November 2001: 5).

Indeed, somewhat unusually, health professionals as well as social workers have now begun to be targeted for criticism in the context of defective child protection practice. An independent review of health professionals' handling of the Lauren Wright case, who died following a blow to her stomach from her stepmother, criticised the health service's response to child protection and joint working. Doctors, it was suggested, must guard against professional arrogance and a 'misplaced belief in their own skills' (in Gillen 2002a). In March 2002 the Carlile review published 150 recommendations aimed at better safeguarding children treated by the NHS in Wales (see Dobson 2002). During spring 2002 a health visitor was also 'struck off' for sub-standard work in relation to child protection. *Community Care* magazine observed: '[S]uch is the status of child protection within the health service that these events, on a scale which would have triggered a major bout of soul-searching had they taken place in an acute sector discipline, have barely caused a ripple . . . [M]any social work professionals have learned to their cost that the health service is often the weakest link in the child protection conference and the area child protection committee' (see the editorial 'Bitter pill for the NHS', *Community Care*, 4–10 April 2002: 5).

The social work/police relationship, the main focus of this chapter, has also been turbulent. An analysis of the perceptions of police officers and social workers is, therefore, important because it may help us to better understand why the relationship has historically been the focal point of ruptures in joint working endeavours (Secretary of State for Social Services 1988; Orkneys report 1992; Gillen 2002b). Perhaps equally important, social work in Britain failed, particularly during the 1980s and 1990s, to properly analyse the historical trajectory and contemporary operational modalities of policing (see, for example, Thomas 1986, 1994). Maybe, during this period, troubling facets of policing were apt to be ignored or neutralised in a discourse blandly centred on 'working together', shared 'professionalism' and combating 'stereotypes'. Just as fundamental was unwillingness to interrogate how social work with children and families was, perhaps, also being remade, in terms of its operations and values, because of the new proximity to policing.

Clearly, social services organisations and the various police forces have many similarities. Both social workers and police officers are created and create their own specific professional discourses and organisational cultures. Both social services and the police bureaucracies were also, throughout the 1990s, subjected to a reconfiguration of their traditional roles and 'ways of seeing' because of the imposition of an aggressive market-driven 'performance indicator' culture (Hall 1998; Adams and Horrocks 1999; see also 'Blair to shake up police culture', *The Guardian*, 17 February 2001). This remaking of social work – and policing – was, for some observers, connected with a more pervasive breaking down of discrete specialisms and professional fragmentation and was identified as evidence of postmodernism (see Carter 1998). That is to say, the blurring of roles and fluid boundaries between professional groups, often perceived as a consequence of multidisciplinary working, was interpreted as reflecting more fundamental societal transformations (Reiner 2000). Given such shifts, Leonard (2000: 106), amongst others, has predicted an acceleration of the 'de-differentiation of expert positions and skill boundaries within state health and welfare organisations'.

The chapter will begin by briefly referring to the emergence of 'child protection' and to research which has specifically focused on the social work/ police relationship. This will be followed by an examination of empirical research, from the Major period, which looks at police officers' accounts of their child protection activity and of how 'working together' is perceived. The remainder of the chapter will focus on joint police/social work units. It will be suggested that there are dangers of professional 'blurring' and risks that social work identities, within these units, may evaporate, or be subject to what is termed voluntary liquidation.

The report into the Cleveland affair (Secretary of State for Social Services 1988: 249–50) had actually recommended the establishment of multidisciplinary 'specialist assessment teams (SATs)' which would consist of an 'approved medical practitioner, a senior social worker and a police officer'.

Towards the end of the 1990s there appeared, however, to be a detectable cooling towards this 'radical' innovation (see, for example, HMIC 1999: 23). An examination of this dimension of the 'working together' paradigm is, however, newly topical because of the re-emergence of the idea that there needs to be a separate, multidisciplinary agency to overview child protection (see Kendall and Harker 2002). The second phase of the Climbié inquiry, for example, explored the idea once again. The suggestion was, however, rejected by the Association of Directors of Social Services (ADSS) because it was felt that there is a 'risk of polarising children in need, and those in need of protection, as two distinct groups when they are on a continuum' (ADSS 2002b). This view was also supported by the former chief social services inspector, William Utting, but others, including the National Society for the Prevention of Cruelty to Children (NSPCC), told the Climbié inquiry that new multidisciplinary child protection teams would improve agency responses (see also the editorial 'No need for revolution', *Community Care*, 9–15 May 2002: 5).

The specific character of the social work/police relationship in child protection is also central importance because of the new social work/police proximity in youth offending teams (YOTs) created following the Crime and Disorder Act 1998 (see Hunter 1999; McCurry 1999a, b; Bailey and Williams 2001). As an HMIC (1999: 3) report has correctly conceded the significance of police forces 'working in partnership' with social services and other associated professionals has been 'brought into sharper focus' on account of these new multidisciplinary teams. Indeed, for the NSPCC, YOTs provide a model for an entirely reconfigured child protection service (see Downey 2002: 36).[1]

The emergence of 'child protection'

In the 1970s, individual police forces were on the margin in terms of responding to the familial harm of children. At a conference of social welfare professionals, held in England in May 1973, James Mounsey of the Lancashire constabulary castigated his audience for failing in 'an important citizen's duty', in that in cases involving the familial harm of children the police were summoned only 'as a last resort' by other agencies. Consequently, he stated, the first time that he and his police colleagues often encountered a child with a 'non-accidental injury' was 'on the mortuary slab' (Mounsey 1975: 127–8). However, by the late 1970s and early 1980s the police were increasingly being integrated into case conference structures (Parton 1985) despite concern from some about the impact of this development on civil liberties (Freeman 1983: 132). More generally, by the mid-1980s the overall thrust of government policy and official circulars was focused on the idea of 'child protection' and on trying to identify or 'target' so-called 'dangerous families' (Dale *et al.* 1986) where abuse was likely to occur and improving the co-ordination of statutory agencies (such as social services, schools, the police).

Some have maintained that approaches such as this, and the emphasis on inter-agency and inter-professional co-operation and co-ordination rest on 'an implicit ideology of neutral, benevolent expertise in the service of consensual, self-evident values' (Challis *et al.* in Eason *et al.* 2000: 356). Thus, from this perspective, 'working together' might be seen as a 'force for conservatism' (Eason *et al.* 2000) because we have an assumption that advanced societies 'face no fundamental structural problems or contradictions, that their problems are merely organisational and interorganisational in character, and that an organisational and interorganisational technology can be created to deal with problems' (Benson in Eason *et al.* 2000: 356).

None the less, in the late 1980s, child-care social workers and police officers gradually began to 'work together' and to conduct joint investigations into the sexual abuse of children, and this prompted controversies connected with investigations in Rochdale, Nottingham, the Orkneys and, of course, Cleveland (Secretary of State for Social Services 1988: ch. 6; Campbell 1988; Bell 1988). However, despite occasional tensions, by the end of the Major period the police were viewed as being 'at the heart of' the inter-professional matrix being mobilised in order to 'protect children' (Department of Health 1995a: 72). More recently the 'refocusing debate' and the introduction of the *Framework for the Assessment of Children in Need and their Families* has reflected a change of emphasis in relation to how best to assess and respond to the needs of vulnerable children (Audit Commission 1994; Department of Health 1995a; Department of Health, Department for Education and Employment, Home Office 2000). None the less, the social work/police relationship remains central in child protection activity (see also Home Office, Department of Health 2002).

Broad overviews of the 'working together' paradigm, featuring both Social Services Departments and the police, have been provided by, for example, Hallett and Stevenson (1980), Hallett and Birchall (1992) and Hallett (1995). A number of research studies are, moreover, available on particular local examples of Social Services Departments and the police 'working together' in the context of child protection. Conroy *et al.* (1990) conducted a study, for the Police Foundation, of a joint initiative which had been set up by the Surrey Constabulary and Surrey Social Services Department. The following year the same team of researchers produced a national survey on joint working between the police and Social Services Departments (Moran Ellis *et al.* 1991). This research comprised a national telephone survey and an analysis of two local schemes. It indicated that, by 1989/90, 74 per cent of Social Services Departments were conducting joint investigations of child sexual abuse with the police (see 'Joint working with police on abuse is now the norm', *Community Care*, 13 December 1990).

Waterhouse and Carnie (1990a, b, 1991) conducted similar research into the response to alleged child sexual abuse in four local authority Social Work Departments (SWDs) in Scotland. Problems were 'uncovered' in inter-agency communication in 20 per cent of the cases analysed. Significantly, in the cases characterised by 'satisfactory inter-agency communication' it was discovered that *'social work deferment to the police* or clear specification which agency was to lead the investigation also contributed to good contact and communication between agencies' (Waterhouse and Carnie 1991: 377, emphasis added). Sanders *et al.* (1996) examined the police role in the management of child protection services in Wales and Parker *et al.* (1996) looked at how eight constabularies policed child sexual abuse in England and Wales (see also Hughes *et al.* 1996; Humphreys 1996; Lloyd and Burman 1996). Davies *et al.* (1998) specifically focused on the training of police officers involved in child sexual abuse investigations and, in the same year, HM's Inspection of Constabulary (HMIC) produced a critical overview of police involvement in child protection (HMIC 1999).

Other research studies, published during the Major period, which examined local Social Services Department/police co-operative initiatives include: Gardiner's (1991) study of co-operative endeavour between Hampshire Social Services Department and the Hampshire Constabulary; Gibbons's (1991) study of a child protection unit housing both social workers and police officers; studies of joint working in central Scotland by Findlay (1991) and Brown and Fuller (1991a, b). Lardner (1992), again in Scotland, studied a child protection unit. Still in the 1990s, Adams and Horrocks (1999), based in West Yorkshire, examined child protection in the context of more general shifts in the organisation of policing (see also Hughes *et al.* 1996; Parker *et al.* 1996; Davies *et al.* 1998; HMIC 1999; Brown and Heidensohn 2000).

All the interviews featured in this chapter were conducted by the author in the mid-1990s in three units, in three different areas of Britain. That is to say, those referred to as 'Whiteley', 'Romley' and 'Killeen' (see Table 1). The names of the localities and the respondents are fictitious, but the brief biographical details, if provided, are the actual details of the respondents. Whiteley was selected for research purposes because it was situated at one end of what might be referred to the 'working together' continuum. This area had the more typical operational model, a child protection unit comprised of police officers only. The constabulary had, however, been castigated by an HMIC report for failing to provide sufficient designated police child protection units within the force area. As we have observed, the report into the Cleveland affair (Secretary of State for Social Services

Table 1 The composition of the three child protection teams

Child protection unit	Composition
Killeen (KCPU)	Social workers and police officers
Romley (RCPU)	Social workers and police officers
Whiteley (WCPU)	Police officers only

1988: 249–50) had actually recommended the establishment of multidisciplinary 'specialist assessment teams (SATs)'. In Romley and Killeen there had been some movement towards this model, in terms of the social work and police elements, in that joint units had been set up. Such units represented, therefore, the operational apex of 'working together' in that here it was literally so in so far as social workers and police officers shared the same office.[2]

The comments of the respondents, often contentious, controversial and robustly expressed, are none the less important because the views of 'front-line staff' rarely find their way into the 'official' discourses on child welfare. Moreover, most research has arguably produced a somewhat sanguine picture of joint working (see, for example, Hughes *et al.* 1996: 43). Here the aim is not to promote a facile social work/good and policing/bad dichotomy. As suggested earlier, strategies of governance and regulation are complex and simplistic approaches are apt to undermine our understanding. The intention is simply to report and critically comment on social workers and police officers' accounts of their jobs and of 'working together'. More fundamentally, in terms of the book's main theme, we shall also see how 'working together' with the police has contributed to the remaking of social work with children and families. Perhaps also important here is the need to bring to the fore the perceptions of police officers who are able to provide a view, albeit often tendentious, from the 'outside' of the remaking of social work with children and families.

Snapshots of joint endeavour during the Major period

Working Together to Safeguard Children (Department of Health, Home Office, Department for Education and Science 1999: 23) asserts that the 'police recognise the fundamental importance of inter-agency working in combating child abuse' and the DI heading the WCPU was very critical of his police colleagues in Cleveland in the mid-1980s. In short, 'it was a total fuck-up, they just pulled out'. In relation to social work and social workers, more generally, he was of the view that:

Like police officers, social workers are good, bad and indifferent . . .
You get some brilliant social workers and they're worth their

weight in gold, but a brilliant social worker is not as common as a brilliant police officer in this line of work . . . Social workers are okay if they're not entrenched in their views, but a lot of them see us as too hard and not comforting enough. The thing is we have to try and make a case stand up in court.

(DI Fearns, WCPU, who has had responsibility for organising all aspects of investigation and training in respect of child protection
in his locality)

Within the WCPU the position of the officers with regard to the 'working together' ethos was put succinctly by a male DC:

We have to work with Social Services Departments because we're obliged to. [However,] it's still police officers doing the job [child abuse investigations], but now social workers will come along.
(DC Stokes, WCPU; see also Hallett 1995: 122)

This was an attitude mirrored in the joint police/social work child protection unit in Killeen.[3] Here all the police officers expressed the view that the KCPU model was a sound one and that the relationships within the unit were good. The senior police officer suggested, however, that his constabulary was *the* lead agency:

Through going out together [on visits to families] the police see the needs of social workers, *but more importantly for us* the social workers see the need from the police side of it. Police officers will always take the statement, and if the social workers need to know things by all means they'll check it out and ask questions. *But the unit is here predominantly to prosecute any offenders and the social workers are here to service the needs of the police* . . . and the Social Work Department.
(DS O'Neill, KCPU, emphasis added)

This somewhat hesitant and convoluted statement pointed to the primacy of the police and an agenda of prosecution within the KCPU. As will be discussed below, this police insight into the 'joint' initiative was also shared by at least one of the social workers in the same unit.

In some instances police officers voiced a certain disregard, even contempt, for their social work colleagues:

Eighty per cent are very good, but 20 per cent only worry about themselves and create hassles. This 20 per cent have what I call 'attitude problems'. Unfortunately, they're not properly educated . . . They're always running to their line managers, saying we don't pass information on to them . . . its like they're running to teacher.

(DC Brown, WCPU)

A colleague added, 'They're often like kids . . . "If I don't get my way I'm not playing".' Another constable described a 'typical social worker' as 'wearing corduroys, with an unkempt appearance, but with their heart in the right place'. He went on:

I had no dealings with social workers prior to this work [in the WCPU] and the training course beforehand. Doing this, I think you get insights into each other's problems: both organisations are clearly pushed to the limits . . . The problem I have with Social Services is that you never seem to get a decision from any individual social worker. I can make a decision, but social workers just seem to look around the room when a decision needs making.

(PC Dee, WCPU)

Such a response may be understood as reflecting some of the 'core assumptions', held by serving police officers, identified by Holdaway (1986). Specifically, ideas about time and modes of decision making (see also, in this context, Hallett 1995: 126). In addition, other comments by police respondents were rooted in particular perceptions about the local population: social workers' 'hearts may be in the right place', therefore, but police officers possessed *the* knowledge about human nature. Social workers were not 'in the real world' (PC Dee, WCPU).

A female PC stated, 'I write down everything they [social workers] say . . . I've found them to be liars.' In contrast, the Whiteley Social Services Department Emergency Duty Team was 'brilliant . . . they get all the shit and get dumped on' (PC Stroud, WCPU). The same constable had clear views on the role of social workers when children were jointly video-interviewed:

The police officer takes the lead in interviews; social workers don't understand them. They are *not* therapeutic interviews, but you get some social workers wanting to spend half an hour saying 'Well done' and 'You're ever so good,' yet the kid just wants to 'rock-'n'-roll' [disclose that abuse had occurred]. They *need* to talk . . . Sometimes I think that they [social workers] don't really want the kid to talk because it [sexual abuse] offends them . . . After the interview as far as I can see they do 'sweet FA' apart from a bit of 'keep safe' work . . . If we get a really nasty case I prefer them [the abused child or young person] to go to Victim Support. Without

VS a lot of them wouldn't stick it out, but VS are brilliant with children . . . I call them 'my families crutch'.

(PC Stroud, WCPU)

Clearly, this view (whilst again pointing to a particular construction of 'time') is one which sought to discredit and delegitimise social work intervention in relation to child abuse within families. Victim Suppport, however, Home Office-funded and controlled and largely staffed by volunteers, was posited as an alternative and malleable 'social work'.

Sanders *et al.* (1996: 88) observed that the 'dichotomy between treatment/therapeutic objectives and investigative/legal objectives' frequently creates a polarity between the police and social services/health colleagues. In Killeen this was, perhaps, illustrated in relation to a planned Health Authority resource. The aim was to establish a 'centre for the vulnerable child': a therapeutic project, which hoped to take referrals from the KCPU. However, for the DS, this was 'a bit fraught with danger':

We have to be very careful whom we pass on [which children] because of the nature of their therapy. They [the therapeutic project] are wanting in as quickly as possible and we have to be careful that evidence is not tainted . . . things might come out in therapy which contradict the statement [the child has made] or else it may appear [in court] that the child has been coached.

(DS O'Neill, KCPU, emphasis added)

This comment, perhaps, indicates that the needs of children were, perhaps, at risk of being entirely harnessed to the needs of the criminal justice system and to bureaucratic imperatives. Furthermore, such an approach would seem to be at odds with the Children Act 1989, which lays down that the welfare of the child should be the 'paramount consideration' (see also Home Office, Crown Prosecution Service, Department of Health, Action for Justice 2001; Valios 2001).

Related to this issue, the social workers interviewed identified a number of tensions with the police presence in the unit in Killeen. One concern focused on the crucial question of whether or not to believe what a child was saying in the context of abuse allegations (see also Hicks and Tite 1998). Here the observations of social work staff also mirror the concerns of respondents featured in Hallett (1995: ch. 5). Two social worker respondents in the KPCU stated that whether or not a child was telling the truth or not was frequently an issue of considerable ambiguity, and this was highlighted by all their professional training and subsequent professional experience. Moreover, if a child was manifestly 'lying', then that, in itself, was perhaps indicative of other factors about the child and its relationship with the rest of the family. However, for the police, only the binary oppositions of 'truth' and 'lies' seemed to exist. If a child did tell 'lies' this, furthermore, often prompted individual police officers to 'take it personally':

> If the police don't believe the child and we do it can be really difficult. You've got to be careful you don't become confrontational with the child . . . The police tend to take it very personally being lied to, I'm used to it . . . The question for me is 'If the child is lying, *why* are they lying?'
>
> (Ms Green, KCPU)

A social work colleague expressed a similar view:

> If they're interviewing a child and they think the child might not be telling the truth [about an allegation of abuse] it's very difficult for them because all their training tells them to approach interviewing in a very confrontational way, yet we know that this is not helpful for the child, who if they're lying are lying for a reason, and it doesn't help to be told 'You're lying.'
>
> (Ms Clinton, KCPU)

One of the social workers in the RCPU also felt that there was a police tendency to seek a resolution of child protection matters in the courts. Thus if the 'evidence was not there' for a criminal prosecution, the police would hope that the civil courts would impose an order. That is to say, the police were less prepared than social workers to seek the non-statutory resolution of child protection issues.

In general, therefore, the police approach to issues of both selection and interviewing 'witnesses' seemed to indicate that certain 'core assumptions' (Holdaway 1986), methods of management and operational techniques characteristic of mainstream and 'traditional' policing were regarded, by the police, as being unproblematically transferable to interventions in connection with child abuse within families.

Some research has highlighted police officers' enthusiasm for multidisciplinary training on child protection (Hughes *et al.* 1996: 28–9; see also Davies *et al.* 1998). However, in Whiteley the five-day joint training course that the constables undertook prior to beginning work in the unit was much criticised, and a particular point of tension with social workers was, it appeared, the issue of 'language':

> It's offensive and patronising to tell people how to talk . . . With certain Social Services Department offices in Whiteley it's as if we are members of a club, but only part-members.
>
> (DC Stokes, WCPU)

They tend to tell us off and pick us up on phrases that we use . . .
You can't even say 'boobs'. I'm forty years old and I get really
pissed off when somebody tells me how to talk . . . Yet it's okay
for them to tell jokes about vicars . . . I don't like that, I'm a
Christian.

(PC Stroud, WCPU)

In this context, given social work's proclaimed value base and the commitment to anti-discriminatory and anti-oppressive practice, the social
workers in the joint units were asked whether this resulted in any tensions,
given what was known about the 'canteen culture' of police forces (see also
Macpherson 1999; Anthias 1999; Reiner 2000). In terms of police attitudes,
one respondent spoke specifically of her experience in the KCPU:

Sometimes I despair – perhaps that's too strong – but there are
things said in here which are discriminatory. They might be just
winding me up or they might not be: for example, the use of the
word 'darkie' a lot . . . yet I don't think it's them [the police officers
in the KCPU] being racially discriminatory. What it is, is their culture. I'm sure if they thought about it they don't really have discriminatory attitudes, but this vocabulary has grown up in the police.

(Ms Clinton, KCPU)

This response, therefore, whilst identifying racist language within the
KCPU went on to excuse it: to explain it away, ease it out of the 'working
together' discourse. Indeed, it might be argued that this approach is part
of the *price* of the joint unit paradigm (and the more general closer working relationship with the police in the context of child protection). Aspects
of police behaviour, perhaps even 'institutional racism', are not contextua-
lised by, for example, previous research on operational policing (see Smith
and Gray 1983; Macpherson 1999; Lea 2000; Reiner 2000). More fundamentally, perhaps, the increasingly close relationship between Social
Services Departments or Social Work Departments and the police, best
illustrated by the joint unit endeavour, may be informed by an implicit
agreement between the police and white social care professionals that
certain aspects of police behaviour – in this instance racist language – are
not challenged, but tolerated, in the interests of maintaining 'working
together' arrangements.[4]

Becoming a 'child protection unit thing': the voluntary liquidation of a social work identity

In the mid-1990s, as the 'refocusing' debate was getting under way, an
editorial in *Community Care* (1–7 June 1995) asserted:

One of the worrying trends in child protection investigations is the growing emphasis on law enforcement. They have become procedure-ridden, and social workers often feel that they act more in the manner of a special constabulary than as carers with a brief to support the child and the family.

This concern about the gradual liquidation of social work and the evolution of a 'special constabulary' can be examined in the joint social work/police units. A female PC, interviewed in Romley, believed that the 'blurring' of social worker/police role critique was 'an insult to social workers'. None the less, locally, the joint unit was a matter of political acrimony. A letter from the Labour chairperson of the Romley Council observed:

> [T]he police and social workers [are] housed in the same building and there appeared to be a blurring of the roles of social workers and the police. This was particularly confusing for our customers [*sic*], who did not understand the different roles of social workers and the police.

None of the social workers, however, felt the criticism that their role and function was becoming 'blurred' was valid:

> It's just prejudice, the stuff about social workers losing their identities and professionalism and becoming more focused on gaining evidence for the prosecution – becoming little social policemen . . . I'm aware of the criticism that the police dominate the social workers, but I put that down to teething troubles . . . All the social workers here are strong personalities, but that wasn't the case when the unit first opened. We are confident about what it is we do, we're not likely to be bullied or intimidated. When the unit first opened there was a particular police officer who was very bullying and a male chauvinist and, I guess, there were a number of social workers who were not, perhaps, very strong in their identity and professionalism, and they did get drawn towards 'police-type' views. One social worker, in particular, started saying, apparently, stuff like 'He put his hands up,' 'He's a bit of a nonce,' and so on. I don't know if this was reflected in their practice, but a certain impression was given . . . things have moved on a hell of a long way since, though.
>
> (Ms Shenton, two weeks in the RCPU)

The same social worker condemned elected council members who opposed the joint unit concept. Thus the Labour group were dismissed as 'all conservative with a small 'c', running from middle-of-the-road to positively fascist' (Ms Shenton, RCPU).

None the less, the DI in the same unit conceded that 'occasionally' the police officers 'helped' social workers by, for example, telephoning local schools to check details about the injuries of children – a task which social workers and not police officers would ordinarily be expected to undertake. Another social worker in the RCPU confirmed that police officers could view Social Services Department files, but this could not be for 'a general rummage' (Mr Barker, a member of the RCPU for eight months).

In Romley, therefore, social workers, sharing the same office as police officers (a former 'safe house' next to the police station) and visiting families together, saw no danger of any 'blurring' and believed – as the lengthy response above makes plain – that their 'professionalism' would be a bulwark against this occurring. In addition, the development of such joint units was not thought to be reflective of wider-ranging and deeper social and political themes. Consequently, one of the social workers believed that joint units revealed nothing about the direction of social work or, more broadly, social policy. In short, for her, the setting up of the RCPU and similar units was merely a pragmatic response to a particular social problem:

> The reason I hope we have these joint teams is simply convenience . . . The job gets done better with less time and energy wasted if we do it together and the outcome is better for the child . . . I don't think, for example, that it has any big implications for social work.
>
> (Ms Pine, six weeks in the RCPU)

One of the police officers in the KCPU believed that there was something of an overlap in terms of the roles of police social workers and police officers:

> I feel sometimes that we give similar advice. On occasions when the unit is really busy and maybe you can't go out with the person who you were out with before – say on a return visit to let a family know what has happened, and two police officers go out together – you can give the appropriate advice a social worker would give . . . Sometimes we [the police] do go out on referrals when there's no need, or there's not enough evidence, or whatever, for any police action so what we're there doing, really, a social worker's job.
>
> (PC Cranmore, KCPU)

Such a remark recalls some of the influential ideas in Alderson (1979; see also Stenson 1993). Indeed, implicit in the apparent ease of movement from police officer to 'social worker' is, perhaps, a certain feigning of expertise and the aim of overcoming 'rigid professional demarcations'. In this context, moreover, social work risks being deskilled and rendered superfluous.

As with their social worker colleagues in Romley, the social workers in Killeen believed that there was no 'blurring' of roles between social workers and the police in the unit. However, in reality, this was not the case in that some degree of blurring was taking place, as is apparent in the following response:

> There's still this thing in society that social workers are here to take your child away and, in some ways, the police are less feared by parents . . . I've actually gone out with one of the other girls [female police officers] on visits [to families] and allowed it to be believed that I was a police officer as well – without actually saying I was a police officer – because if I said I was a social worker it would merely antagonise the situation . . . The case I'm thinking about involved a very aggressive lady who hated social workers. She'd been a product of the care system herself and her son had been in care. It was only for about half a day that she didn't know that I was a social worker and that was because she was bouncing and raving and saying that she wanted to kill them and 'do time' . . . If it did have any impact on how she related to me it was short-lived.
>
> (Ms Clinton, KCPU)

Clearly, this comment made it plain that in some instances parents did not know *who* was in their home making observations and assessments about their standards of parenting. Here the social worker *became* a police officer. In joint units the likelihood that this blurring may be used as a 'technique' with 'difficult families' could be increased because of the closeness of the relationship between the 'two services'. The blurring – in the above instance more a willed liquidation of the social work role and the switching of the social worker into a police officer – is not, however, simply explicable in terms of the duplicity of individual social workers. It is, perhaps, rooted in the evolution of social and economic relationships in a 'market society' (Taylor 1999; Crowther 2000). That is to say, given the scale of material hardship and the associated shattering of communities, certain areas, particularly inner-city locations, are unwelcoming to the 'caring professions', perhaps especially social workers inquiring about the welfare of children. For social workers on 'problem visits', therefore, the presence of the police may also help offset a certain sense of foreboding, even fear (Department of Health 2001e). As one social worker commented:

I actually feel much safer going out with a police officer. People realise that they have the weight of the law behind them and that to assault a police officer is almost worse than assaulting a civilian: whereas people wouldn't hold back in going for me, they might hold back in going for a police officer . . . The girls [female police officers] are very brave and they're not easily intimidated, whereas personally I am. They're confident if there's a potentially violent situation, so I feel a lot more assured actually going out [to visit families] . . . I think you're able to do the work properly if you're less concerned about your own personal safety. In times in the past when I've been a social worker going into the homes of children on supervision orders, for example, parents have been angry and hostile and clearly didn't want me there – they're in the middle of a life crisis, they've got a lot going on in their lives and they're ready to go for you. I don't feel safe in those situations, and I think that's an issue for social workers generally.

(Ms Clinton, KCPU)

Returning to the question of social workers' identity becoming fused with that of the police officers in the KCPU, one social worker felt that she had, in fact, ceased to be a social worker:

I'm not really a social worker; I'm not a police officer . . . I'm this 'child protection unit thing' now.

(Ms Polster, KCPU)

This particular social worker was the most enthusiastic about the KCPU of the social workers interviewed and she felt that social workers in the unit had 'more in common with them [the police] than with some of the colleagues in my profession'. Central to her engagement with children who might have been abused was the gathering of 'clean evidence'.

As far as I'm concerned *I'm servicing the police*. I'm trying to get a child to tell me what happened, so there's a weight of evidence for my police colleagues to go and confront a guy with . . . Quite clearly, I'm offering my skills to the police as a means of investigation. I'm pretty far on in terms of talking to children, I've got an awful lot to learn yet, but what I've got I'm offering to the police.

(Ms Polster, KCPU, emphasis added)

Such an understanding of social work may be entirely logical in terms of the function of joint police/social work units. Social work intervention risks being simply annexed to the central police task: the gathering of evidence to ascertain whether there is enough available to charge a 'suspect'.

Moreover, within this framework, the assembling of 'clean evidence' is prioritised, and the discourse and practice centring on the familial harm of children risk becoming entirely criminalised. This criminalisation of the discourse of child protection can, moreover, also be viewed alongside the more encompassing criminalisation of child welfare discourses, referred to earlier in the discussion of aspects of the LAC scheme.

Conclusion

Ward and Peel (2002: 223), in their examination of inter-agency approaches in child welfare, have argued that, for collaborative working to be successful, five elements are essential: an identified purpose, consensus, choice, reciprocity and trust. In this chapter, focused on a small research study undertaken during the Major period, it is clear that these 'essentials' were largely absent. More fundamentally, the interviews at the heart of the chapter indicate that police officers, irrespective of the organisational form in which they are located for child protection purposes, are apt to want to retain a leadership role and are frequently reluctant to form a 'partnership of equals'. On occasion, problems in joint working appeared to be compounded because officers (sometimes embattled and inward-looking) felt marginal within their own constabularies (see also the editorial, 'Met's step and start', *Community Care*, 11–17 July 2002: 5). More fundamentally, the continuing closeness of the social work/police engagement in the context of 'child protection' continues to evidence the need for more critical analysis of this relationship.

The whole notion of 'working together' is now embedded in the wider social work and social care discourse of the New Labour administration in Britain (Eason *et al.* 2000; Webb and Vulliamy 2001). More specifically, in focal ideas about 'joined-up thinking' and 'joined-up working' (see, for example, Department of Health 1998d; see also Payne 2000). This is reflected at the level of practice in, for example, the emphasis on multidisciplinary teams in the emerging Care Trusts and, as we shall see in Chapter 8, in the philosophy underpinning the Connexions agency (Department for Education and Employment 2000a). It also relates to some of the ideas associated with the 'corporate parenting' of 'looked after' children. However, the suggestion here has been that there is often a failure to interrogate what these rhetorical assertions about multidisciplinary working actually amounts to in terms of the micro-politics of 'joined up' endeavours.

In terms of the future, we are advised that teaching for the new social work degree is to stress that social workers 'must work effectively with other professionals for the benefit of those who rely on social services' (Department of Health 2002b). Significant here, however, must be the fostering of a reflexive willingness to try and critically comprehend other disciplines and the social processes that underpin joint working paradigms.

Elsewhere in the Department of Health literature we are told that the 'reform of social work training' must also be concerned about 'building up social workers' confidence in their own skills and knowledge' so that when they 'operate in multi-professional settings' they will be 'confident and flexible' (SSI 2001: 8). This chapter suggests, however, that a sense of confidence in the social work role – its purpose and its values – is clearly vital.

Part II will now identify and examine some of the main developments which have taken place during the period of the New Labour administrations.

Part II

THINGS CAN ONLY GET BETTER?

New Labour and social work with
children and families

> I say to those who are undermining our public services: if you're
> on the side of the people who use public services, you should also
> be on the side of the people who work in public services as they
> make the reforms vital to those services. If you're on the side of
> the pupil, you should be on the side of the teacher. If you're on
> the side of the citizen, you should also be on the side of the police.
> If you're on the side of the patient, you should also be on the side
> of the nurse, the doctor, the hospital staff.
> (From Tony Blair's speech on public services at the Centre of Life,
> Newcastle, 25 January 2002)[1]

Perhaps also 'If you're on the side of the looked-after child, you should
also be on the side of the social worker'? Clearly, social workers remained
conspicuously absent when the Prime Minister commended the work of
public service workers. Indeed, this omission reflects the Blair administration's rather lukewarm approach to social work. However, this is not to
argue that the two New Labour governments have ignored social work, or
unambiguously worked to promote its demise. The Major period witnessed
many changes in social work, and the transformations which were
prompted – in practice and organisational structure – have accelerated
under the Blair administration's 'modernisation' agenda (Department of
Health 1998d). The government is, for example, committed to introducing
a new three-year programme of undergraduate social work training. None
the less, social work remains in crisis (Unison 2002).[2] Perhaps most notably
in terms of inability to recruit a sufficient number of staff. As a DoH
review of the operation of the Children Act 1989 wryly observed, 'The

maintenance of skill levels is clearly dependent on posts being filled. Whilst a filled post may represent variable skill levels, an unfilled post represents a zero skill level' (Department of Health 2001f: 88). In this context the low morale of those currently in post is clearly significant (Jones 2001).

Specifically within the sphere of social work with children and families, political, professional and managerial energies are being devoted to embedding post-qualifying accreditation and to the implementation of the *Framework for the Assessment of Children in Need and their Families*. Local Social Services Departments also continue to make often creative use of monies released under the QP initiative (Department of Health 1998b). Quality Protects was launched by the government in September 1998 and the Children's Services Grant supports it. In October 2000 the programme was extended from three to five years, with funding increased from £375 million over three years to £885 million over five years. The aim, according to the Department of Health, is to 'focus on the most vulnerable and disadvantaged children in society – those looked after, those in the child protection system and other children in need' (Department of Health 2002d). The Children Act 1989 has also been substantially amended by the Care Standards Act 2000, the Children (Leaving Care) Act 2000, the Carers and Disabled Children Act 2000 and the Criminal Justice and Courts Service Act 2000.

However, Bill Jordan (2001: 527) has observed that 'social work in the UK seems to be faring worse under a Labour government than it did during eighteen years of Conservative administrations'. The second Blair administration appears intent on divesting local authority social work of key areas of operational responsibility (see also Jordan with Jordan 2000; Butler and Drakeford 2001). Social work with children and families hardly featured in, for example, the consultative paper *Supporting Families*, published during the period of the first Blair administration (Ministerial Group on the Family 1998). In addition, there have been successful attempts to restrict local authority social work's entry into many of those new zones being created for engagement with 'disadvantaged' children and families. A number of initiatives introduced in the area of children and family services have, for example, been located outside local authority Social Services Departments. These include the Sure Start programme (Glass 1999; see also Wilson 2002), the Children and Young People's Unit, and the £70 million Children's Fund (Holman 2000). In England, in October 2001, the inspection of childminding services was also taken over by the Office for Standards in Education (Taylor 2001; Rickford 2001). The children's residential care sector is now also gradually diminishing as a proportion of local authorities' market share (Kirkpatrick *et al.* 2001), although the situation does not, of course, reflect that in the United States (Fabricant and Burghardt 1992). However, following the general election of 2001, a number of Ministerial statements have focused on the need to involve the private sector more in public services, and this suggests that children's residential care is likely to be more drastically reconfigured in the future. More drastically, the setting up of Children's Trusts, announced in the government's spending review in August 2002, could result in children's services being removed altogether from the control of local authorities (Downey 2002).

Youth justice has also been placed under the auspices of the Youth Justice Board (YJB) and multidisciplinary Youth Offending Teams (YOTs). As a result 'services for children in trouble' have been separated from 'mainstream children and families services' (Goldson 2000: 256). This separation was, moreover, emphasised in *The Children Act Now: Messages from Research* (Aldgate and Statham 2001) which failed even ro refer to young offenders (see also Howard League 2002a). Equally important is the YJB's aim of ideologically distancing itself from the former approach and its dominant liberal ethos. So, for example, one edition of the YJB's glossy monthly newsletter contained a grotesque photograph of a grinning social worker wearing a bullet-proof vest (see 'Rotherham gets results, Texan-style', *Youth Justice Board News* 8, June 2001: 5). Significantly, he is on a visit to the United States, learning how things are done 'stateside'.

The Blair government has also introduced a 'star rating system' for Social Services Departments, with a number of councils awarded 'zero stars' being subjected to visits from 'performance action teams' which include consultants from large corporations ('Private sector to help four worst councils', *The Guardian*, 30 May 2002). Developments such as this reflect, perhaps, a New Labour view that local authority social work is too closely associated with 'old' Labour enclaves and 'old' and 'unsuccessful' ways of intervening in the lives of children and families (see also 'Blair "seeking a fight" with council staff', *The Guardian*, 13 July 2002). Equally striking is the lack of radical discontinuity between the administrations of Major and Blair in relation to how socially and economically marginal children and families are apt to be regarded and constructed. More generally, as Martin Jacques (1998: 3) has observed, for 'all the hyperbole, it is the continuities rather than the ruptures that characterise the Blair era' (see also Newman 2001: 1–2). Indeed, more than a hint of 'authoritarian populism' (Newburn 1996) continues to underpin, for example, a number of the youth justice policies of the second Blair government. We have also seen the continuing criminalisation of the discourses of child welfare. The Prime Minister himself, when in opposition, was apt to display a somewhat reductionist approach to child welfare in general, in that the success of a particular policy was tested against its potential ability to reduce crime (see, for example, 'Nursery school for all children can cut crime, claims Blair', *The Guardian*, 9 September 1993). Likewise, the former Home Secretary, Jack Straw, remained convinced that 'the roots of criminal behaviour are planted in childhood' (Straw and Anderson 1996: 2). He went on, therefore, to devise a range of measures to 'break the excuse culture' which was allegedly failing to adequately deal with young offenders. The Crime and Disorder Act 1998 provided for an array of mechanisms, such as Child Safety Orders, Antisocial Behaviour Orders and local Child Curfews, which enable local authorities to regulate the spatial movement of errant youthful bodies (Walsh 2002; see also 'Council tenants warned to keep child footballers off the street', *The Guardian*, 28 August 2000).

More generally, within New Labour's discourse on child welfare, actual social work practice 'remains entirely shadowy, portrayed either as anxious monitoring or decisive protection, or even as tough enforcement, but never as sensitive, aware, dialogical and flexible negotiation' (Jordan 2000: 125). However, perhaps it is with the continuing use of the LAC materials and the new Framework that a vision of practice emerges from the shadows. The next chapter will, therefore, critically focus on the Framework and on its contribution to the remaking of social work with children and families.

Across a wider canvas, and partly influenced by some of the social policy departures of the former Clinton administration, a new 'toughness' is evident in terms of responses to those who refuse to accept their parental 'responsibilities'. In New Labour's second term we have seen the threat of Child Benefit being withdrawn from parents whose children play truant and the introduction of legislation which would permit the withdrawal of Housing Benefit for those responsible for 'antisocial behaviour' (see 'Cabinet split over plans to stop Benefits', *The Guardian*, 29 April 2002; 'New Benefit crackdown', *The Guardian*, 30 April 2002; see also the contrasting editorials 'We should link Benefits to duties', *The Observer* 5 May 2002, and 'Blair should know better', *New Statesman*, 6 May: 6–7). Furthermore, in spring 2002 a mother was sentenced to sixty days' imprisonment because she had failed to ensure that her children attended school ('Judge refuses to bail mother of truants', *The Guardian*, 16 May 2001; see also Garrett 2001). Moreover, these policies and developments provide, it will be suggested in Chapter 6, part of the ideological backdrop for the New Labour approach to child adoption. In a more pervasive sense, a reinvigorated 'tutelage' orientation to intervention in the lives of children and families is apparent in New Labour's 'parenting orders' and, as will be highlighted in Chapter 8, in the whole Connexions approach to working with young people (Donzelot 1979; see also 'Back to school for abusive parents', *The Guardian*, 24 March 2001).

The arrival in government of New Labour appeared to herald a more sensitive approach to issues associated with 'race' and ethnicity and this was soon reflected in the decision to set up an inquiry examining the circumstances surrounding the murder of Stephen Lawrence (Macpherson 1999). The Race Relations (Amendment) Act 2000 should also have an impact on how Social Services Departments relate to black and ethnic minority families (Home Office 2002a). However, running counter to these developments has been failure to adequately respond to the emergence of 'xeno-racism' (Fekete 2001). Indeed, key New Labour measures targeted at asylum seekers and refugees increasingly contribute to the growth of racism being encountered by many children and families (Cohen 2002). Although, in opposition, New Labour opposed the more oppressive aspects of Conservative asylum legislation, the Immigration and Asylum Act 1999 'went even further in restricting rights' (Sales 2002: 471). Specifically, in relation to children and families, an editorial in *Community Care* (28 March–3 April 2002: 5), observed that this measure is a 'heinous piece of legislation' which places many 'children and families outside the welfare state' and that it is another example of 'institutional racism' in Britain (see 'Children to be dispersed in plan to cut asylum seekers', *The Guardian*, 28 May 2002, and the editorial 'Divisive monitoring', *Community Care* 18–24 July 2002: 5). Furthermore, the Children's Rights Alliance has submitted a report to the United Nations Committee on the Rights of the Child which has asserted that the Blair government's treatment of refugee children and asylum seekers is 'inhumane and degrading' (in Valios 2002: 28). The Nationality, Immigration and Asylum Act 2002 permits the Home Office to confine asylum seekers, like nineteenth-century workhouse residents, to special centres where they will be denied access to the NHS and mainstream schooling. In Chapter 7, whilst chiefly focusing on Irish children and families, it is maintained that social work's engagement with issues of 'race' and ethnicity remains conceptually flawed because of the dominant tendency to view the world solely in terms of 'black' and 'white' identities.

5

SOCIAL WORK AND THE THIRD WAY

The Assessment Framework, New Labour and more new 'tools' for social work with children and families

A national standardised assessment model, introduced by the Blair administration in April 2000, is central to the remaking of social work with children and families. This chapter will, therefore, analyse and comment on aspects of the *Framework for the Assessment of Children in Need and their Families* (Department of Health, Department for Education and Employment 2000) and accompanying materials. Chief amongst the latter are the contributions in *The Child's World: Assessing Children in Need – Reader* (Department of Health 2000b); *Assessing Children in Need and their Families: Practice Guidance* (Department of Health 2000c); *The Child's World: Assessing Children in Need – Trainer Modules* (Department of Health, NSPCC, University of Sheffield 2000) and *The Family Pack of Questionnaires and Scales* (Department of Health, Cox and Bentovim 2000).[1]

In this chapter the intention is to provide part of the context for the evolution of the Framework by referring to some of the comments of its primary definers and a number of the relevant background documents which have been issued by the Department of Health since the late 1980s. This will be followed by an articulation of the new assessment paradigm featured in the Framework. It is then suggested that the Framework can be more fruitfully understood not only in terms of previous policy documents and earlier technologies of intervention related to child protection and, more broadly, child welfare; it also needs to be more expansively perceived, fixed and located as it relates to other elements in New Labour's faltering political 'project'. In this context it is further suggested that the trajectory of Welfare policies in the United States is relevant (see also Harris 2002). The chapter will conclude by examining, in more detail, two facets of the Framework which are of major importance for social workers' micro-engagements with children and families. First, the Framework's theoretical preoccupation with an ecological approach to social work assessments. Second, the significance of the questionnaires and scales which accompany it.

The Framework is issued under section 7 of the Local Authority Social Services Act 1970, which requires local authority social services to act under the general guidance of the Secretary of State. As such the Framework lacks the full force of statute, but will be complied with 'unless local circumstances indicate exceptional reasons, which justify a variation' (Department of Health, Department for Education and Employment, Home Office 2000: preface). In practical terms, therefore, the Framework is likely to be viewed as mandatory. Making clear the centralising consequences of this development, it is emphasised that the 'protocols, procedures, forms and methods of record keeping and practice resources of all authorities and agencies should be consistent with the Assessment Framework and the principles which underpin its use' (Department of Health 2000c: 114). The Framework was implemented in England in April 2001 and in Wales in April 2002.

Importantly, the new assessment model 'builds on and supersedes' *Protecting Children: a Guide for Social Workers undertaking a Comprehensive Assessment* (Department of Health 1988; see also Department of Health, Department for Education and Employment, Home Office 2000: preface). A good deal of the 'thinking' which underpinned this so-called 'orange book' has, however, been 'incorporated' into the Framework (Department of Health, Department for Education and Employment, Home Office 2000: preface). Despite the redundancy of this, heavily criticised, earlier assessment schedule it is still of some use, we are advised, because it continues to 'contain a useful set of questions' (Adcock 2000: 63). However, some of the problems associated with it are acknowledged, since inspections and research have shown that the guide was 'sometimes followed mechanistically and used as a checklist, without any differentiation according to the child or family' (Department of Health, Department for Education and Employment, Home Office 2000: preface). As we shall see later, however, this comment seems somewhat paradoxical, given the proliferation of questionnaires and scales introduced as part of the Framework's package of materials. The defective 'orange book' was designed to provide an assessment framework for long-term planning in families where there are child protection concerns, but the new Framework is intended for use in the initial assessment of all 'children in need'. Consequently, it is 'embedded' in the revised *Working Together to Safeguard Children* (Department of Health, Home Office, Department for Education and Employment 1999) and for the 'first time children who are referred to a social services department will be assessed according to the same dimensions irrespective of their presenting needs' (Department of Health 2000a: 74; see also Cantwell 2000).

A prominent factor prompting the introduction of the Framework is connected with 'research findings regarding the . . . narrow focus on child abuse . . . in terms of social workers' understanding of the assessment task and outcomes for children and families' (Howarth 2000: 19). As a result, family support services have been slow to evolve and there has been an 'emphasis' in practice 'on a reactive social policing role with services targeted at children at risk of significant harm' (Howarth 2000: 20; see also Department of Health 2000a). As 'a result of the focus on child protection' the assessment of children and families became 'characterised as assessment of the risk of abuse' (Rose 2000: 30). The influential *Child Protection: Messages from Research* (Department of Health 1995a), together with other reports (such as that of the Audit Commission 1994), are also revisited in order to remind us that 'a negative environment, particularly one of low warmth and high criticism is likely to be more damaging in the long term than an isolated incident of physical abuse' (Howarth 2000: 21; see also Campbell 1996, 1997; Cleaver *et al.* 1999; Hunter 1999). Another key theme, which has prompted the Framework's evolution, is identified as the growth of 'mutually exclusive' family support and child protection services (Howarth 2000: 24). In addition, there is the lack of emphasis on environmental and familial networks and the practice failure to integrate a child's, or family's, 'strengths' as well as 'difficulties' into assessments. Much of this is familiar, of course, in terms of the refocusing debate which took place in Britain and the United States in the 1990s (see also Kamerman and Kahn 1990; Waldfogel 1998, 2000). The key departure here, however, is that a new assessment paradigm, or 'conceptual map' (Howarth 2000: 26), has been created to enable social workers to address their theoretical and practice shortcomings. In brief, the approach to the assessment of children and families needed to be 'altered and *modernised*' (Howarth 2000: 24, emphasis added).

As will be suggested later, the Framework is firmly rooted in New Labour's 'modernising' project and needs to be responded to by taking into account this social and political dimension (see also Department of Health 1998d). Specifically – and prior to exploring the 'conceptual map' – it should also be emphasised that the Framework is a 'central plank' of the Blair administration's Quality Protects (QP) programme which is concerned with improving children's services (Department of Health 1998a, b, e; Hutton *et al.* 2000). The Framework will, we are advised, assist local authorities in meeting one of the QP objectives to 'ensure that referral and assessment processes discriminate effectively between different types and levels of need, and produce a timely service response' (Department of Health 1999a: preface; see also Department of Health 2000a: ch. 8).

Reading the map

Importantly, it is acknowledged that a 'child's needs cannot be fully described unidimensionally, but require more than one axis or domain' (Sinclair and Little 2002: 134). The Framework is, therefore, pictorially represented in the form of a triangle or pyramid, with the child's welfare at the centre, and this 'conceptual map' is to be used by social workers and other social care professionals to 'understand what is happening to children in whatever setting they may be growing up' (Department of Health 1999a: 26). The social work assessment of children and their families should take into account 'three systems or domains whose inter-actions have a direct impact on the current long-term well-being of a child' (Rose 2000: 32). These are identified as a child's developmental needs, the parenting capacity and the family and environmental factors (Department of Health, Department for Education and Employment, Home Office 2000: ch. 2). Figure 1 indicates how each of these domains is subdivided into a series of other dimensions.

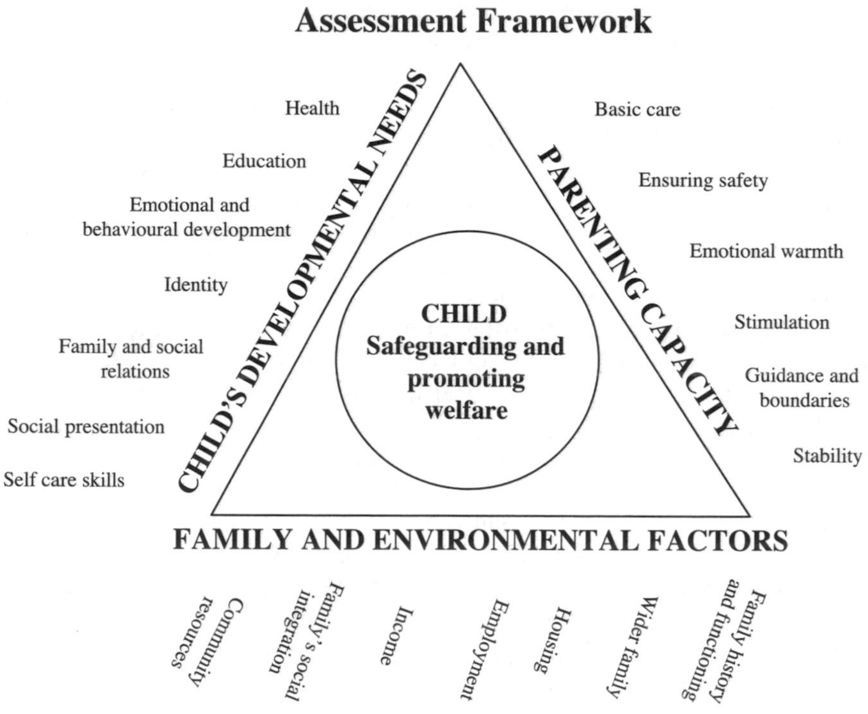

Assessment Framework

Health
Education
Emotional and behavioural development
Identity
Family and social relations
Social presentation
Self care skills

Basic care
Ensuring safety
Emotional warmth
Stimulation
Guidance and boundaries
Stability

CHILD'S DEVELOPMENTAL NEEDS
PARENTING CAPACITY

CHILD
Safeguarding and promoting welfare

FAMILY AND ENVIRONMENTAL FACTORS

Community resources
Family's social integration
Income
Employment
Housing
Wider family
Family history and functioning

Figure 1 The Framework for the assessment of children in need and their families

The 'child's developmental needs' domain inherits those dimensions formulated by the creators of the LAC system discussed in Chapters 2–3 (see also Parker *et al.* 1991; Ward 1995a). It is notable that, within the discourse centred on the new Framework, there has been a slight shift in terms of how particular aspects of children's development are regarded, and this is apparent in a brief but revised and less prescriptive discussion of 'social presentation' (Ward 2000b: 131; see also Kilroe 1996). None the less, both LAC and the Framework retain a similar view of the world in that current social and economic relationships are uncritically perceived and presented as providing an unquestioned foundation for familial dynamics and interpersonal relationships. Thus, in the new Core Assessment Record, part of the Framework materials, we find that social workers are expected to ascertain whether young people respect 'the concept of ownership' (and to blandly answer Yes/No) (question B13). In the context of an assessment of 'parental capacity', social workers are also expected to assess whether the 'parent teaches respect for the law' (question B32). Similarly, workers are directed to find out whether parents provide guidance on 'good manners' (question B28). Elsewhere, and somewhat cryptically, in the same document, it is asked whether the parents' relationship with 'those in authority' is generally 'harmonious'? (question B29). Whilst sharing aspects of the same ideological disposition as the LAC enterprise, the new Framework will, however, be used with a far larger group of service users. In this sense these authoritarian questions are, perhaps, rendered even more significant. Such questions can also be associated, as will be suggested later, with a new political fixation in both Britain and the United States on the personal behaviour of welfare recipients.

More explicitly, in terms of a narrower professional discourse, the 'domain' preoccupied with 'parental capacity' (see also Jones 2000) is heavily influenced by *Child Protection: Messages from Research* (Department of Health 1995a) and particular attention is directed, in the associated commentary materials, to families where there are issues related to mental illness, drug and alcohol misuse and domestic violence (Cleaver 2000; Rose and Aldgate 2000; see also Cleaver *et al.* 1999). Importantly, and perhaps taking into account firmly grounded criticisms that social work assessments have tended to centre on and scrutinise only mothers, the new Framework, on occasion, also stresses that fathers need to be adequately assessed (Department of Health, Department for Education and Employment, Home Office 2000; see also Garrett 2001).

The third 'domain', concerned with 'family and environmental factors' is included because of the way in which 'individuals and families internalise social and cultural norms so that the world outside lives in the minds and feelings of those within the family' (Stevenson in Rose 2000: 25). This psychodynamic approach to environmental factors is, however, coupled with a more subtle and emphatic understanding of the impact of poverty on parenting and family functioning (see also Garrett 2002). This fresh acknowledgement, within the official discourse of child-care social work, is striking and welcome and sets the Framework apart from child-care policy documents produced by the previous administrations of Thatcher and Major (see, for example, Rose 2000: 31–2; Rose and Aldgate 2000: 14–15). Clearly, this is connected with New Labour granting 'permission' for poverty to be discussed, and this aspect of the Framework will be returned to later (see also Blair 1999). More generally, 'inclusive practice' features as a recurring motif throughout the Framework (Department of Health, Department for Education and Employment, Home Office 2000: 26–7). This construct is connected with New Labour's 'social exclusion' discourse and seeks to provide a new theoretical anchorage for a range of child-care social work issues previously formulated in terms of 'anti-discriminatory', 'anti-oppressive' or 'anti-racist' practice. Marchant and Jones (2000) and Dutt and Phillips (2000), therefore, usefully seek to relate the use of the 'conceptual map' to social work interventions where questions of disability, 'race' and ethnicity are central. In the latter contribution we also find a welcome, but still problematic, discussion of white ethnicities.

Finally, the cartographers are intent on stressing that their endeavours are driven by the 'evidenced-based approach' (Gray 2000: 8; in this context see also Webb 2001). The 'body of knowledge available to those who struggle with today's problems of child care is still rudimentary compared with the physical sciences; but is far and away greater than we could have called upon in the past' (Parker in Gray 2000). As a consequence of these developments the Framework is, therefore, 'grounded in knowledge' (Rose and Aldgate 2000: 1). Knowledge is then defined as 'theory, research findings and practice experience in which confidence can be placed to assist the gathering of information, its analysis and the choice of intervention in formulating the child's plan' (Rose and Aldgate 2000: 1). This epistemological orientation also sets out to partition off 'ideology' and to combat potential ideological contamination: 'It is . . . important not to confuse theory with ideology. Work with children and families has sometimes been subject to fashionable ideologies, which may dictate the style of work adopted. Ideological approaches should never get in the way of ethical and professional practice' (Rose and Aldgate 2000: 1; similar remarks are found in Ward 2002: 26). As with its LAC predecessor, therefore, the social work practice which the Framework seeks to promote risks becoming merely a composite set of technical assessment tasks driven by 'evidenced-based knowledge' about 'what works' (see also MacDonald and Roberts 1995; Hodgkinson 2000; Taylor and White 2001; Sanderson 2002). Furthermore, this flattened practice, bolstered by a positivistic conception of social sciences, would seem to exist above and beyond 'ideology'. A social work, in fact, for the 'Third Way' (see also Jordan 2000).

New Labour, new Framework

The Framework is firmly embedded in New Labour's vision for Britain and this is apparent in the materials associated with the new assessment paradigm. The vocabulary of the Blair administration is found throughout and, more fundamentally, various authors are keen to stress where the Framework features in the government's social and economic plans. Jack (2000b: 50), for example, excitedly proclaims:

> The Labour government, elected in 1997, has recognised the importance of tackling child poverty and has set itself the ambitious target of eliminating it altogether by the year 2019. Economic policies have been introduced: the national minimum wage, New Deals to improve employment opportunities, tax credits for working families, children and child care increases to child benefit which are designed to lift 700,000 children out of poverty within three years. Other programmes include Sure Start for early child care and Action Zones to pilot ways of improving education, health and communities. [See also Gray 2000.]

Comments such as these invite us, therefore, to widen the analytical net and to locate the Framework within New Labour's 'project' and to engage with some of New Labour's focal ideas and preoccupations – particularly those related to the 'new paternalism' and 'social exclusion'.

Chantal Mouffe (2000: 113) has maintained that 'New Labour represents the clearest example of the "Clintonization" of European social democracy'. Indeed, the uncritical use of phrases such as 'Welfare dependency' in DoH literature on social work with children and families in Britain (Aldgate and Statham 2001: 236–7) reveals how a number of New Labour's focal ideas on the welfare state have been influenced by the 'welfare reforms' of the 1990s Clinton administration in the United States. Walker (1999: 683), for example, has also argued that the Blair administration 'resonates with a potpourri of US influences' (see also Fairclough 1999; King and Wickham-Jones 1999; Swanson 2000; Deacon 2000; Prideaux 2001; Prince 2001; ADSS 2002b; Newburn 2002; Nixon *et al.* 2002). Furthermore, there is evidence of US corporations materially penetrating into areas of social care which were previously the responsibility of the welfare state in Britain (see, for example, 'UK elderly care plan run by US "cheats"', *The Observer*, 10 November 2002). Significant in terms of dominant *ideological* approaches, however, is what has been termed the 'new paternalism'. This has been defined as social policies 'aimed at the poor that attempt to reduce poverty and other social problems by directive and supervisory means'. Consequently, programmes based on these policies 'help the needy but also require that they meet certain behavioural requirements . . . These measures assume that the people concerned need assistance but that they also need direction if they are to live constructively' (Mead 1997: 3). The suggestion here, therefore, is that a British variant of the 'new paternalism' can be understood to provide part of the ideological backdrop for the new Framework.

An important element in this approach to Welfare lies in the notion that there exists a 'contract' between government and governed. Central here is 'conditional' Welfare and this is most emphatically illuminated, of course, in relation to the work obligations with the New Deal (see also Etzioni 1995: 82–3; Peck 1998). However, 'conditional' Welfare is now also apparent in other Welfare domains where behavioural compliance is required before aid from the state becomes available (see also Smiley 2001). This applies, for example, to access to council housing (conditional on behaviour) and maternity grants (conditional on child health checkups) (Powell 2000: 47; Vaux 2000; Young 2000; see also 'Free childcare – if young mothers return to school', *The Guardian*, 22 February 2001). It has also been proposed that access to unemployment benefits might become conditional on a claimant's willingness to receive tuition in literacy and numeracy (see 'Claimants face cuts for shunning 3 Rs', *The Guardian*, 5 December 2000).

Significantly, this 'new politics of conduct' (in Deacon and Mann 1999: 426) and the focus on personal behaviour is now played out, as we shall see in Chapter 8, in an array of micro-engagements and is framed by, for example, parenting orders and envisaged encounters with a seemingly benign phalanx of personal advisers, mentors, 'Big Brothers and Sisters' and so on (Ministerial Group on the Family 1999). This reinvigorated drive to remoralise and to create a network of supervisory and tutorial relationships can also be viewed as rooted in what Deacon (2000: 11) has aptly dubbed 'Anglicanised communitarianism' (see also Donzelot 1979; Campbell 1995b; 'Blair's moral crusade', *The Observer*, 2 September 1999; Butler and Drakeford 2001). These developments and transformations – to many, evidence of 'governmentality' (Rose and Miller 1992) – are also enmeshed in discourses and practices centred on children and families. More precisely, they are frequently preoccupied with the 'parenting capacity' of socially and economically marginal parents, often mothers (Milner 1993; Krane and Davies 2000; Scourfield 2000; Turney 2000; see also Smart 1992). This is reflected in the discourse on the Framework in, for example, Jack's (2000b: 44) uncritical references to research in the United States, which is entirely focused on 'neglectful' mothers. The same fixation can also be seen in the introduction of so-called 'parenting orders'. In reality, these are more akin to *mothering* orders, with the YJB revealing, in summer 2002, that 81 per cent of the 3,000 parents starting a 'parenting programme' between spring 1999 and the end of 2001 were, in fact, female (Youth Justice Board 2002b).

Utilising aspects of the dominant discourse on parenting for explicitly political purposes, Hoghugi and Speight (1998: 295) have also made a rather chilling plea for governments to become the 'parents of society' arguing that:

> Governments should be regarded as the parents of society. A 'not good enough parent' of a government will show a general lack of care for the whole population, will put its own interests first, will discriminate against some of its 'children' in favour of others and will react excessively punitively when some of its children mis-behave. A 'good enough parent' of a government will truly care for all its children and will seek to promote their welfare, while still being firm and fair in applying sanctions for unacceptable behaviour. [See also Taylor *et al.* 2000.]

It becomes, therefore, increasingly difficult to extricate specific technologies of social work intervention, such as the new Framework's 'parenting capacity' construct, from more encompassing political and cultural pre-occupations and projects. In brief, despite the claims of the Framework's formulators, 'ideology' and 'ethical and professional practice' (Rose and Aldgate 2000: 1) cannot, as they suggest, be so easily separated out.

Examining New Labour approaches, Gail Lewis (2000: 268) has identi-fied the 'reinscription of the heterogeneous family as the core unit of a stable, law-abiding and responsible citizenry'. The Framework acknowl-edges that there can be a 'diversity of family styles' (Rose and Aldgate 2000: 9) and that there should be, as we have seen, 'inclusive practice' (Department of Health, Department for Education and Employment, Home Office 2000: 26–7), but this is rendered somewhat shallow when else-where New Labour advises that 'marriage is still the surest foundation for raising children' (Ministerial Group on the Family 1999: 4). Similarly, within social work's discourse, and despite the Framework's rhetorical pro-motion of social inclusiveness, exclusionary new classifications and typolo-gies for 'problem families' are being reforged (see Cleaver and Freeman 1995: 51–3; Eisenstadt 1998; Steele 1998). Meanwhile, many asylum seekers continue to be excluded or corralled and 'dispersed' (London 2000; Parker 2000; Cohen 2002; Sales 2002). Below, however, we will seek to examine, in more detail, the idea of 'inclusive practice' which is inseparable from the Framework's new approach to assessment.

Examining 'inclusive practice'

The idea of 'inclusive practice' relates to one of New Labour's main orga-nising principles, combating 'social exclusion'. This concept can be traced to 'the somewhat surprising synthesis of social Catholicism and republicanism in contemporary France' and – from the late 1980s in Britain – to its deployment by the Commission of the European Union (Byrne 1999: 8). By the mid-1990s, 'social exclusion' had become central to New Labour's 'social justice' discourse (Commission on Social Justice 1994). As a result, both within social work and elsewhere, the term 'social exclusion' and the activities of the New Labour administration's Social Exclusion Unit are apt to dominate discussions concerning the conceptualisation of, and response to, poverty (see Barry and Hallett 1998; Dowling 1999; Bowring 2000). Washington and Paylor (1998: 335), for example, have argued that 'the developing usage of the concept of social exclusion offers social work an opportunity to establish a professional focus which can be used in practice throughout the member states of the European Union'. However, 'social exclusion', which is part of the theoretical bedrock of the new Framework, needs to be approached more warily and with a degree of reflexive caution.

'Social exclusion' has, for example, been criticised for seeking to mask poverty and the related questions of income and wealth distribution. Ruth Levitas (1996) has criticised this 'new hegemonic discourse' since 'social divisions which are *endemic* to capitalism' are presented as 'resulting from an *abnormal* breakdown in social cohesion' (emphasis added). The concept also raises issues connected with low pay, because work is unproblematically perceived as *the* mechanism of social inclusion. Indeed, not 'since the workhouse has labour been so fervently and singlemindedly valorised' (Hall 1998: 12; see also 'New Deal to scour streets and set homeless to work', *The Observer*, 26 November 2000).[2] Levitas (1996: 18) contends, for example, that to 'see integration as solely effected by paid work is to ignore that fact that society is – and certainly should be – more than a market'. Lister (1997) has levelled a similar critique at 'social exclusion' and its fetishism of work which is, in reality, often low-paid and associated with few employment rights (see also Fitzpatrick 2001; Haylett 2001b). More generally, the New Labour vision 'treats differences as matters reconciled through the normal and "normalizing" identity of being a wage earner. Wage work is no longer reserved for white, able-bodied, males: anyone can (and should) be a breadwinner' (Powell 2000: 48). These criticisms should, perhaps, have particular resonance among social workers, who daily engage with people excluded from the labour market because of ill health, disability, age, caring responsibilities or discriminatory employment practices.

Key interventions by New Labour figures have also highlighted a new element in 'social exclusion', which might be referred to as the 'social exclusion gene'. That is to say, there exists the notion that 'social exclusion', entirely detached from economic processes, can be transmitted from generation to generation. At the launch of the Social Exclusion Unit,

Prime Minister Blair, for example, asserted: 'Social exclusion is about income, but it is about more. It is about prospects, networks and li, chances. *It is a modern problem likely to be passed down from generation to generation*' (in Alcock 1998: 20, emphasis added). Alistair Darling, the former Social Security Secretary, echoed these sentiments when he claimed: 'Many of these people live on the worst estates. They will die younger; *statistically there is a good chance their exclusion will pass on to their children*' (Darling 1999, emphasis added). This reflects, moreover, some of the discredited ideas which underpinned the 'cycle of deprivation' theory in the 1970s (Haylett 2001a: 361–2; Deacon 2002; Denham and Garnett 2002). A conceptual relationship which is further emphasised by the government's intention to 'break the cycle of disadvantage, to stop it *being transmitted through generations*' (Department of Social Security 1999: 5; see also Jordan 1974).

Given this focus on the *reproduction* of 'social exclusion', it is, of course, hardly surprising that the Blair government has placed so great an emphasis on motherhood (see Haylett 2001b). More specifically, on seeking to prevent, in the vocabulary of New Labour, 'teenage pregnancy'. In 2000, therefore, the Blair administration appointed 150 teenage pregnancy co-ordinators to 'drive thorough the campaign to cut teenage pregnancies by 50 per cent by 2010' (Department of Health 2000d). Indeed, pregnant teenagers remain significant in the government's narrative on account of their alleged readiness to pass on their 'misconceived negativity about education, training and employment' (Colley and Hodkinson 2001: 341; see also Haylett 2001a, b). More fundamentally, New Labour's orientation can also be interpreted as part of a more historically rooted approach to poverty that seeks to locate the cause of poverty in the behaviour and failings of the poor themselves (see, for example, Bosanquet 1895; MacNicol 1987; Murray 1990; Dean 1992; Robinson and Gregson 1992; Rodger 1992; Mann 1994; Haylett 2001a). Equally important, on account of the narrowness of the dominant social and political vision, this lends itself to an ecological approach to social work theory and practice.

The ecological approach to assessments

The ecological approach is emphasised throughout the Framework, especially in the commentary by Jack (2000b), and the prominence given to this particular theoretical orientation gels with New Labour's 'Third Way'. Thus it can be argued that trying to view the Framework through the, somewhat opaque, lens of the 'Third Way' provides some insight into its theoretical preoccupations and subtexts. More fundamentally, this approach is rooted in the understanding that we cannot treat 'cultural texts', such as the new assessment materials, as if they are 'hermetic or pure', since 'representations are linked to wider social forms, power and public struggles' (Giroux 2000: 355).

As Stuart Hall (1998: 9) argues, the 'Third Way' remains New Labour's bid to capture and define the 'big picture'. On one level its central claim is merely 'the discovery of a mysterious middle course on every question between all existing extremes' (Hall 1998: 10; see also Navarro 1999; Neocleous 1999; Jameson 2000; Powell 2001). However, the 'Third Way' does have one key defining feature, and that is bound up with the perception of 'globalisation' (see also Bauman 1998; Sivanandan 1998/9; Khan and Dominelli 2000). New Labour has brought 'a sweeping interpretation of globalisation, which it regards as the single most important factor which has transformed our world' (Hall 1998: 11). Within this dominant discourse, 'globalisation' is constructed as a 'self-regulating and implacable Force of Nature' and the global economy becomes 'in effect like the weather' (Hall 1998: 11; see also Atkinson 2000: 223). As a result, the government set about 'vigorously adapting society to the global economy's needs, tutoring its citizens to be self-sufficient and self-reliant in order to compete in the global market place'.[3] The framing strategy of New Labour's economic repertoire remains, however, essentially the neo-liberal one: 'the deregulation of markets, the wholesale refashioning of the public sector by the New Managerialism' (Hall 1998: 11; see also Clarke and Newman 1997; Rose 1999).

Turning to social work, ecological approaches have historically been concerned with crime and 'juvenile delinquency' and are rooted in American urban sociology, particularly the 'Chicago school' which was prominent during a period stretching from the 1920s to the 1940s (Jack 2000b: 42; see also Shaw and McKay 1969; Giddens 1989: 555–64). The main aim of social work, within this theoretical orientation, is to 'strengthen the adaptive capacities of people and to influence their environments so that transactions are more adaptive (Germain and Gitterman in Payne 1997: 146; see also Maluccio *et al.* 1986: ch. 1). Here, therefore, the 'emphasis on *adaptiveness* illustrates the way ecological theories assume fundamental social order and play down possible radical change' (Payne 1997: 146, emphasis added). Importantly, this 'adaptive' orientation, strongly influenced by US writers, receives a new articulation in the Framework and it strongly underlies its approach to social work engagement with children and families (Cochran and Brassard 1979; Luster and Okagaki 1993; Seita 2000; see also Jack and Jordan 1999).

Clearly, social work assessments must take account of environmental factors, but the specific way in which such factors are constructed suggests that 'communities' are, as the 'Third Way' would have it, powerless in the face of 'globalisation'. The various references to US texts concerned with ecological approaches in Jack (2000b), for example, are revealing in that the titles imply that social workers should not concern themselves with actually promoting the qualitative social and economic transformation of communities. Instead, social work is merely to aid and facilitate *individual* strategies and survival plans. In short, the chief aspiration of social workers and others involved in 'joined up' endeavours is simply to create *Urban Sanctuaries* (McLaughlin *et al.* in Jack 2000b: 56) where children have the opportunity to *Escape from Disadvantage* (Pilling in Jack 2000b: 56) and to be successful in *Overcoming the Odds* (Werner *et al.* in Jack 2000b: 56). Within this 'adaptive' paradigm 'social workers have a role to play in developing social capital in *deprived* communities' (Jack 2000b: 48, emphasis added). Such neighbourhoods might then be 'poor, but decent place(s) to live' (Garbarino and Kostelny in Jack 2000b: 48). In short, social work is merely to aid people as they hunker down behind the rocks as the fiery tides of globalisation wash all around them.

The notion of social capital is, as Jack (2000b) makes plain, associated with the Framework's ecological perspective. Social capital, 'paralleling the concepts of financial capital, physical capital and human capital', is 'embodied in relations among persons' (see Coleman 1988: 120). Its specific 'attributes' consist of 'trust, commitment to others, adhering to social norms and punishing those who violate them' (Bowles 1999; see also Jack 2000a, b). Significantly, social capital is increasingly prominent in policy discourses in the United States, but has been criticised for its 'conceptual ambiguity' and for its proponents' failure to recognise and explore the proposition that although social capital might 'facilitate intra-group co-ordination, by identifying group identity it promotes inter-group hostility' (Durlauf 1999: 4; see also Morrow 1999; Etzioni 2001).

More fundamentally, it might be argued that the Framework's theoretical attachment to social capital reflects, as suggested earlier, the major impact which US theory and practice appear to be having on child welfare policy in Britain. Jack (2000), for example, highlights the range of community-based interventions being carried out in the United States (see also Glass 1999). However, when evaluating the impact of such programmes and asserting that similar initiatives are likely to be appropriate in a British context, it is also important to view the plethora of US programmes, targeted at children and families, in the context of other, more embracing 'Welfare reform' policies and modalities of intervention. As observed previously, such programmes and schemes 'for the regeneration of moral community, commitment and connectedness' are frequently linked with the 'new paternalism' and they often have a coercive and punitive component (see Rose 1999: 488). Moreover, changes in federal law, particularly Clinton's 'Welfare reform' flagship – the Personal Responsibility and Work Opportunities Act 1996 – have had enormous detrimental consequences for many children and families using (or now prevented from using) social and health-care services in the United States

(Handler 2000; McGowan and Walsh 2000; see also 'A million parents lost medicaid, study says', *New York Times*, 20 June 2000).[4]

Back to the toolroom

Having put in place aspects of the wider context of the new Framework, the final part of this chapter will narrow the focus once again in order to comment on *The Family Pack of Questionnaires and Scales* (Department of Health, Cox and Bentovim 2000) which accompany it. These 'tools' are comprised of the Strengths and Difficulties Questionnaire, the Parenting Daily Hassles Scale, the Home Conditions Scale, the Adult and Adolescent Wellbeing Scales, the Recent Life Events Questionnaire, the Family Activity Scale and the Alcohol-Use Scale.

The 'conceptual map', outlined earlier, sketches in the contours of the terrain which is viewed as relevant when assessing children and families. The Family Pack, constantly referred to and highlighted in the Core Assessment Record, fits uneasily alongside this new cartology and some of its values, but has been designed 'to provide *objective*, structured information that will help practitioners approach with greater confidence complicated issues' (Ward 2000b: 136, emphasis added). The questionnaires and scales 'widely used in psychology and psychiatry' were, moreover, found to be 'helpful', even 'useful', when piloted in five Social Services Departments in 1998/9 (Department of Health 2000c: 118). They can be used 'following a process of familiarisation, but do not 'require any formal training'. These 'tools' will, however, provide 'a clear evidence base for judgements and recommendations' (Department of Health 1999a: 70). Elsewhere, it is confided, a little glibly, that: 'Good tools cannot substitute for good practice, but good tools can achieve excellence' (Department of Health 1999a: 66).

The questionnaires and scales, also referred to as 'instruments', are interesting on various levels and a number of brief observations can be made. First, we are constantly advised that social workers in the piloting authorities found them 'easy to administer and of immediate benefit' (Department of Health, Cox and Bentovim 2000: 4), yet what is oddly jarring – and perhaps disingenuous, given the Framework's 'evidence-based' discourse – is the lack of evidence. No data are furnished in respect of social workers, or service users' receptiveness to these 'instruments', only the occasional pithy anecdote (see Department of Health, Cox and Bentovim 2000). Second, the importation of these 'instruments' into the social work assessment of children and families may represent a shift towards a more positivistic and psychiatry-led orientation. Perhaps of particular note, in this sense, is the attachment of the 'instruments' to methodologies, which seek to 'screen' for emotional and behavioural disorders via 'scoring' techniques. So, for example, with the Strength and Difficulties Questionnaire 'the scales can be scored to produce an overall score that indicates whether a child/young person is likely to have a significant problem. Selected items can also be used to form subscales for Pro-social Behaviours, Hyper-activity, Emotional Symptoms, Conduct and Peer Problems' (Department of Health, Cox and Bentovim 2000: 16). Here the concern must be about potentially pre-emptive and inaccurate diagnostic labelling, particularly in a wider social context – with its battery of Antisocial Behaviour Orders and child curfews – so primed, and alert to a lack of 'pro-social' behaviour in certain groups of children and young people (see Coppock 1996; James and Jencks 1996; James and James 2001). Historically, the 'psy complex' (Rose 1985) – which these questionnaires and scales represent the ascendancy of – has also been enmeshed in more embracing discourses centred on crime and social disorder (see Birlson 1981: 86). The search for 'criminogenic' tendencies remains, as argued throughout this book, bound up with policies directed at young people in contact with social services. Significantly, during the piloting of the Strengths and Difficulties Question-naire 'over half the children assessed scored above the cut-off indicating a problem disorder' (Department of Health, Cox and Bentovim 2000: 16). The risks of this happening are, moreover, multiplied within a discipline where 'psychiatrists come to diagnostic decisions quickly and direct their attention to confirm their hypotheses' (Birlson 1981: 75; see also Rose 1985, 1989).

Third, the tone of the 'tools' and their accompanying commentary might be viewed as insulting and patronising to the children and families using social services. We are advised, for example, that 'even when there are crises there are times when professionals are consulting with each other and carers or children are waiting. Appropriately presented, a question-naire can help carers or children feel they are still active partners, and that the professionals are still listening' (Department of Health, Cox and Bentovim 2000: 5). Perhaps the notion that a questionnaire can be simplis-tically inserted into social work intervention in this way also highlights the separation of the designers from practice. Moreover, such comments risk seeming to infantilise parents and other carers. Problems are compounded by the language used in the various 'instruments'; for example, some of the questions featured might 'seem daft' in terms of what is asked about 'the kids' (Department of Health, Cox and Bentovim 2000: 12). One wonders what these 'experts' would deduce if the language featured in forms designed for their use, or that of their families, addressed them and impli-citly envisaged, constructed and *fixed* them in this way. Related to this, the Family Pack might be perceived as being at odds with an 'inclusive' orien-tation in that it continually hints at an entrenched class prejudice. So, for example, the Home Conditions Assessment includes a check for 'stale cigarette smoke'. The Family Activity Scales, in a manner suggestive of the activities of Beria's NKVD, is supposed to include 'information about the cultural and ideological environment in which children live' (Department of Health 1999a: 72). Turning to rural pursuits, it also asks whether the family have recently attended a 'county show' or 'fete' (Department of Health, Cox and Bentovim 2000: 24, 40).[5] Neither of these is a leisure activity which can be convincingly associated with life for many children and families in Britain's inner cities. Both, however, are activities which help to conjure up the social milieu of the designers of such forms. A further criticism must also relate to the fact that young people under eleven years of age are not even permitted to self-evaluate with the Strengths and Difficulties Questionnaire because 'parents' reports of their children's emotions and behaviours are usually more reliable than those of children themselves' (Department of Health, Cox and Bentovim 2000: 16).

Fourth, a good deal of the research which is marshalled in order to substantiate the validity and utility of the 'instruments' is unsatisfactory. References to underpinning research for the Adult and Adolescence Wellbeing Scales date from the 1970s and early 1980s. Similarly, research for the Recent Life Events Questionnaire and Family Activity Scale is from the mid-1980s. The fact that it was conducted in the 1970s and 1980s does not, of course, in itself invalidate the research, but it is somewhat surprising that more recent research is not deployed. Furthermore, parts of the research foundation, such as that which informed the development of the Parenting Hassles Scale, is also questionable in that it involved only mothers (see Crnic and Greenberg 1990). Fifth, running as a thread throughout the *Family Pack* is a fixation with the time in which it will take to complete each questionnaire and scale – normally within ten minutes. Along with the new time limits introduced under Qualith Protects to regulate assessments, this suggests that a new time discipline is being constructed for social workers' micro-engagements with children and families (see also Harvey 1990: ch. 4). This has potentially major implications for the *process* of social work and might also be viewed as a dull echo of more pervasive cultural trends centred on what Virilio (1997) has identified as the tyranny of unrelenting acceleration (see also White 1998a).

Finally, and again related to shifts in the process of social work with children and families, these 'tools' illuminate the fact that social work activity is increasingly being contained by a plethora of pro-formas. This is, of course, reflected in the materials associated with the LAC system and the Young Offender Assessment Profiles (ASSET) developed by the Centre for Criminological Research at the University of Oxford (see also Poster 1990). Once again, this trend appears to mimic dominant social work orientations in the United States (Early 2001; Graybeal 2001). Specifically in relation to the Framework, there are potentially far-reaching implications in terms of how the various 'instruments' and 'tools' will come to be used and deployed. In the New Labour world of social work with children and families, will managers begin to ask questions, in professional supervision, about the quantities of questionnaires and scales completed? Similarly, will these managers want to know about particular 'scores' achieved by individual children and families? Will 'scores', or assessments derived from questionnaires and scales, begin to feature in child protection case conference reports, and will professionals begin to use these 'instruments' to calibrate risk? Will judges and magistrates begin to seek from social workers the 'certainties' which 'hard' data appear to provide? More fundamentally, these schedules and checklists are likely to contribute to the shaping of new Welfare 'subjects', new professional subjectivities and to a potential 'emptying out' of social work relationships (see also Lash and Urry 1999: 15).

Conclusion

Clearly, the new Framework, produced by 'leading professionals in the field' (Hutton 2000) and heavy with 'symbolic capital' (Bourdieu 1991) is significant in that it is the first 'official' standard assessment model intended for use in the initial assessment of all 'children in need' under the Children Act 1989 (see also the discussion in Moss *et al.* 2000). The new model embedded in current British and US social welfare discourses will have consequences for children and families and it will have a major impact on child-care social work's theoretical foundation and operational modalities. In the late 1980s it was contended that social work was 'an invisible trade' (Pithouse 1998) and the aim of the Framework and similar procedural documents is, in part, to render the activity more visible and controllable.

Relating our discussion to the LAC system examined earlier, we can see that the Framework's main piece of documentation, the Core Assessment Records, are similar 'in concept the LAC Action and Assessment Records' (Ward 2000b: 136). The rather alienating format of the AARs is retained, and this will be of some concern, given the critique mounted against the AAR 'concept' by many social work practitioners and academics, children and young people (see Knight and Caveney 1998; Shemmings and Shemmings 2000: 94). Indeed, superficially the package of Framework materials is similar, in terms of presentation and format, to the welter of research and promotional materials which appeared when the Department of Health introduced the LAC system (see Parker *et al.* 1991; Corrick *et al.* 1995; Jackson and Kilroe 1996; Ward 1995a; Jackson 1998). However, even though it is argued that LAC was 'a remarkable piece of work' (Rose 2000: 30) and the Framework seeks to develop the LAC approach to assessment, the contributions connected with the new assessment paradigm are also markedly different. Despite some of the similarities – and the problems identified, particularly with the so-called Family Pack – the documentation associated with the new Framework suggests a somewhat more pluralistic project, which is less strident, less uptight and less intent on regulating and policing its ideological boundaries. The 'learning materials development group' (Department of Health 2000b: 9–11), for example, appears to be a broader coalition than the close-knit, insular group responsible for the LAC materials. In addition, issues connected with disability (Cotson *et al.* 2000; Marchant 2000; Marchant and Jones 2000), 'race' and ethnicity (Dutt and Phillips 2000) are addressed in a much more convincing and sensitive way.

Specifically in relation to the scales and questionnaires, it is important to recall that social work, because of its, often uneasy, relationship with the 'psy complex' (Rose 1985) has always had a professional interest in checklists (see Richmond 1917). In some respects, therefore, the Framework and its associated practice materials can be interpreted as merely remodelling more historically rooted 'instruments' of social work practice. None the less, child-care social workers in Britain – beleaguered, bewildered and reinforced by small platoons of recruits from Canada, South Africa and elsewhere – should, perhaps, be asking searching questions about the entire Framework endeavour. The 'excitement' (Department of Health, NSPCC, University of Sheffield 2000: 3) of its designers needs to be momentarily tempered and the new paradigm situated in an expansive social and political context.

The next chapter will examine a further aspect of New Labour's drive to 'modernise', or remake, social work with children and families. More specifically, the initiative to relocate child adoption at the heart of social work with children and families.

6

AN 'EYE-CATCHING INITIATIVE'

New Labour and child adoption

Attempts were made to introduce adoption in the late nineteenth century, but it was not until 1927, following the Adoption of Children Act 1926, that child adoption was legally recognised in England and Wales (Teague 1989; Lowe 2000). Since then reports and legislation have refined policy and professional practice. Moreover the contours of the debate on adoption have been shaped and defined by more embracing political projects and preoccupations. Case law has had an impact, so also – particularly more recently – have 'cases', or 'stories', which have received media attention and reflected social workers' alleged deficiencies in relation to adoption.

The aim of this chapter will be to chart the Blair government's attempts to 'reform' the law on child adoption. This has been a key element in the government's child welfare programme and is contributing to the remaking of social work with children and family. The chief focus will be on the *Prime Minister's Review of Adoption*, which was published as a consultation document in July 2000 (Performance and Innovation Unit 2000). This was followed by a White Paper, *Adoption: a New Approach* (Department of Health 2000e), in December the same year, and the publication of the Adoption and Children Bill in March 2001. The first half of the chapter will refer to the cultural, historical and political context of New Labour's interventions (see also Lowe 2000). This will be followed by a critical examination of some of the key themes detectable in the New Labour approach.

The wider cultural significance of child adoption

The wider public and cultural significance of child adoption inescapably informs how social work relates to the issue. Indeed, in the late twentieth and early twenty-first centuries child adoption has featured prominently in social and cultural discourses. Two New Labour MPs, for example, both birth mothers, were reunited with children – now adults – whom they were separated from through adoption many years earlier (Sone 1996). Films, television documentaries and literature have evinced an interest in the issue. So, for example, Mike Leigh's (1997) award-winning film *Secrets and*

Lies was centrally concerned with child adoption. Meanwhile, in Hollywood, the 'off-the-shelf symbol of stardom is an adopted baby' (Birkett 2002). In Britain, a BBC *Panorama* programme, screened in late 1999, somewhat tendentiously examined adoption and was followed by a more balanced series of documentaries, *Love is not Enough: the Journey to Adoption*, screened in autumn 2000. Jackie Kay's (1991) wonderful poems, featured in *The Adoption Papers*, were rooted in a preoccupation with a child adoption and its emotional consequences. In the early months of 2001 the 'story' of the Kilshaws and a so-called 'Internet adoption' dominated the media (see 'Controversy rages over the twins sold to highest bidder', *The Guardian*, 17 January 2001).

Clearly, the adoption of children will always command a measure of public attention because it touches on a host of substantial and emotive issues centred on, for example, the rights of parents versus the rights of the state (Fox Harding 1991): social constructions of 'childhood' and 'children' at particular moments in history (James *et al.* 1998); how we arrive at notions such as 'good enough parenting' (Adcock and White 1985); how societies are economically structured to enable some parents to cope with the financial costs of children and not others (Bebbington and Miles 1989); sexual orientation and parenting (Sandland 1993); the commodification of children and new markets in child welfare (Van de Flier Davis 1995; Katz 2000; Kirkpatrick *et al.* 2001); neo-colonial practices and how the richer West relates to the 'Third World' and to parts of the former Eastern Bloc (Lowe 2000: 332–3). The discourse of child adoption in the United States, Britain, Ireland and elsewhere has also been bound up with 'race' and how it should be addressed in terms of the placement of children (Cohen 1994; Gilroy 1994; Kirton 1996, 2000; Garrett 2000a, b, c, 2003a; Solinger 2000; Thoburn *et al.* 2000).

The current interest in child adoption – perhaps particularly fascination at the reunion of adopted children with their birth mothers – might also be perceived as reflecting more than the private concerns of specific individuals and could be interpreted as being rooted in more profound and existential questions early in a new century. One might point, for example, to postmodernism's scepticism about 'grand narratives' and related interest in the 'self' and 'identity' (see, for example, Hall 1990, 1992a; Hall and du Gay 1998; Rose 1998). The demise of the Soviet Union and the ending of the Cold War have, of course, also led some to suggest mistakenly that we have reached 'the end of history' (Fukuyama 1992). As overarching material and interpretative structures are said to have disappeared, or been diminished, and life is characterised by increasing uncertainty the adopted person's search for authenticity – for 'roots', for a 'real' sense of self – can carry more general cultural resonance and meanings (see also Schechter and Bertocci 1990; Feast and Howe 1997).

More prosaically, governments in both the United States and Britain continue to exhibit an itching preoccupation with child adoption. In his final State of the Union address President Bill Clinton felt the need to boast that adoptions were 'up by 30 per cent' (Clinton 2000, see also PIU 2000: 64). Similarly, Prime Minister Blair, at a loss because New Labour was inexplicably becoming 'somehow out of touch with gut British instincts' observed, in a leaked memo, that the 'adoption issue worked well' and that it might be politically expedient to trigger a series of other 'eye-catching initiatives' which were 'entirely conventional in terms of their attitude to the family' (see 'What the memo tells us about Tony Blair's style of leadership', *The Guardian*, 18 July 2000). For both Clinton and Blair, promoting a populist child adoption agenda was, therefore, perceived as potentially electorally advantageous, and both administrations have been active in producing policy documents, or legislation, on the issue.

Earlier attempts at 'reform'

Historically, politicians have frequently endeavoured to get 'a grip' on what have been viewed as unsatisfactory adoption procedures (see PIU 2000: 31). For the Conservative administrations of the 1990s, adoption services were fundamentally flawed because social workers were contaminated and driven by 'political correctness' (see Hopton 1997; also Barber 1993). This tendentious judgement was, however, rooted in related preoccupations and projects centred on: the promotion of 'family values' (see Morgan 1999); concern about a growing 'underclass', or – in the words of Charles Murray – a 'new rabble' (Murray 1994; see also MacNicol 1987; Murray 1990; Robinson and Gregson 1992; Rodger 1992; Mann 1994); the political aim of reducing public expenditure, privatising key parts of the public sector and incrementally undermining the ability of local authorities to provide services; the grudging acceptance that Britain was a multiracial society, but – importantly – one which had no further need to interrogate questions associated with 'race' and racism.

In the summer of 1993 media and political attention focused particularly on the case of James and Roma Lawrence, whose application to adopt had been rejected by Norfolk County Council because, it was claimed, of their lack of understanding of 'race' issues (see also Clark 1993). Significantly, in terms of the construction of the case, James was white and Roma was Asian. The Prime Minister, John Major, asserted that he was not 'interested in trendy social theories, only in good homes for needy kids' (see 'Adoption "trendies" attacked by PM', *The Guardian*, 14 July 1993). In November 1993 a White Paper *Adoption: the Future* was published which was presented by Ministers as representing a 'commonsense' approach to adoption, with less emphasis being placed on the 'race' of children and adopters (Department of Health, Welsh Office, Home Office, Lord Chancellor's Department 1993; see also Department of Health and Welsh Office 1992). Elements within the media interpreted the political 'spin' associated with the launch of the White Paper as a move to ban social workers from preventing transracial adoption (see, for example, the editorial 'Happy families: political correctness should be kept out of adoption', *The Times*, 4 November 1993). However, despite political and media representations, no British legislation has ever 'banned' social workers from transracially placing children. Consequently, charges of 'ethno-dogma', occasionally levelled within academic discourse, have also been somewhat misplaced in terms of social work practice with children and families (Gilroy 1994).

In March 1996 the Department of Health published a draft Bill and during the consultation period emphasis was placed on child adoption as an alternative to single parenthood (see 'Adoption law aims at single mothers', *The Guardian*, 25 March 1996). Perhaps, as *The Guardian* suggested, 'It was not difficult to unearth a motive: unmarried mothers cost the state £9 billion in social security. What better wheeze than to transfer this cost to childless middle-income couples desperate to adopt and more than ready to bear the full cost of children.' It was concluded, however, that the draft Bill was 'not nearly so Neanderthal as speculation suggested' (see the editorial 'A child's rights are paramount', *The Guardian*, 29 March 1996). Indeed, beneath the political 'spin' frequently associated with child adoption was a range of mooted changes, which were welcomed by child welfare professionals. Greater emphasis was to be placed on the rights of children in the adoption process (see also Selwyn 1996). The Children Act 1989 establishes that the welfare of the child is the 'paramount consideration', but the principle did not, at that time, feature in adoption legislation in England and Wales. Thus there were plans to introduce a 'paramountcy' principle into new adoption legislation. The Bill, however, ceased to progress prior to the general election in May 1997 (see also 'Adoption Bill halted amid Tory jitters', *The Observer*, 25 August 1996). The Children (Northern Ireland) Order 1995 (see Kelly and Coulter 1997) and the Children (Scotland) Act 1995 did, however, introduce changes.

Social dynamics and adoption

Over the last quarter of a century significant changes have taken place in relation to the social dynamics underpinning the process of adoption. First, on account of the contraceptive pill, social liberalisation and the decline in stigma associated with births to 'unmarried mothers', the number of children being adopted in England has decreased from approximately 20,000 each year in 1970 to 4,100 in 1999 (PIU 2000: 10). The most drastic decline has taken place in respect of babies, that is, children under the age of twelve months: in 1968 12,641 babies were adopted (51 per cent of all adoptions), but only 195 babies were adopted in 1998 (4 per cent of all adoptions) (in Lowe 2000: 319). In short, adoption is now more likely to involve children in public care – or 'looked after' – under the Children Act 1989 who are older, have been at the centre of child protection concerns, or have disabilities or other special or complex needs (see Department of Health 1998f: para. 9; Lowe 2000). Many of these children will have been removed, on a compulsory basis, from their parent(s).

Second, unlike in the past, there is now greater openness in the adoption process (Baran and Pannor 1990; Ryburn 1994; Department of Health 1999b: ch. 5). This approach had been passionately advocated by Ellen Wilkinson, the Labour MP, in the parliamentary debate on the Adoption of Children Bill in 1926 (*Hansard*, vol. 192, col. 952, February 1926). More recently, change in this area has been prompted by the gradual acknowledgement, on the part of mainstream professional opinion, that 'openness' is important in relation to the 'identity needs of adoptees' (Kirton 2000: 108). The retreat from secrecy was also driven by the demands of adoptees who wanted to find birth relatives (see also Campbell *et al.* 1991). In an influential study, Triseliotis (1973: 1) examined the experience of adoptees who searched for biological parents. At the time, he observed that Scotland and Finland were 'the only countries in the Western world where an adopted person can obtain from official records information that could lead to the tracing of the original parents'. The Children Act 1975, however, gave adopted people over the age of eighteen years the right to apply for access to their original birth certificates. In Scotland, the right to information had been provided under the Scottish Adoption Act 1930.

Birth mothers have also pressed for greater openness in adoption (Brodzinky 1990; Bouchier *et al.* 1991; Howe *et al.* 1992; Wells 1993; Logan 1996). Furthermore, the Natural Parents Support Group, an organisation of birth mothers, is lobbying Parliament for a public inquiry to look into the injustices which occurred during the years of mass adoption in the 1950s and 1960s (see Rickford 2000; also Campbell 2000). Some attention has also begun to focus on the marginalisation of birth fathers in the adoption process and in research on adoption (Clapton 1997). More generally, the greater 'openness' has resulted, in some instances, in 'contact arrangements' between the child and birth family *after* the adoption has taken place (Dutt and Sanyal 1991; McRoy 1991; Siegel 1993; Beek 1994; Stone 1994; Mullender and Kearn 1997; Lowe 2000: 326–9). Moreover, the Adoption Act 1976, as amended by the Children Act 1989, required the Registrar General to set up an Adoption Contact Register to enable adopted people to contact their birth parents and other birth relatives. Related to these developments is an increasing awareness of the significance (and inadequacy) of post-adoption services (Hughes and Logan 1995).

Third, today adoptions are much more likely to be contested by birth parents (see Ryburn 1992; Mason and Selman 1997). Furthermore, in this context, it has been observed that 'studies which have looked at the outcome of contested cases found no instance of an application for adoption being refused' and that this 'must occasion unease' (Department of Health 1999b: 122). Finally, a likely growth area in relation to the adoption of babies is that associated with the globalisation of adoption – inter-country adoption (Ngabonziza 1988, 1991; Triseliotis 1991; Duncan 1993; O'Brian 1997/8; Department of Health 1998f: paras 50–4; Groothues et al. 1998/9; Lowe 2000: 332–4). A Private Member's Bill resulted in the Adoption (Intercountry Aspects) Act 1999, but this legislation is still to be fully implemented. However, following the publicity generated by the attempted 'Internet adoption' by a Welsh couple – the Kilshaws – of American twins, the Act is now more likely to be soon fully operational (see also Department of Health 2000e: 34).

Following the general election in May 1997, pressure for adoption 'reform' continued (SSI 1997; Morgan 1998). Central here was the continuing charge that there was 'an anti-adoption culture in adoption departments and agencies' (Alibhai-Brown 1999; see also Engel 1999; 'Carey urges easier adoption laws', The Guardian, 12 May 2000). Again reflecting the ideological convergence between the Major and Blair administrations, the Home Secretary, Jack Straw, called for more adoptions of babies born to 'young unmarried mothers' (see the editorial 'Clutching at straws: teenage mums are made scapegoats', The Guardian, 27 January 1999). Related to these interventions, the government was also, of course, intent on cutting the social security payments of lone parents (see Smith 1999; 'Blair's new tough line on single mothers', The Observer, 1 June 1997; 'Blair aims to make single mums work', The Guardian, 2 June 2000).

Paul Boateng, when Junior Minister at the Department of Health, attacked social services in a way similar to his Conservative predecessors (see Valios 1998). He was particularly concerned about an alleged social work fixation with 'same race' placements, the age of potential adopters, their social class and whether or not they smoked. This, despite empirical evidence published by British Agencies for Adoption and Fostering (BAAF) which highlighted the fact that these alleged preoccupations were not apparent in terms of social work practice in the area of adoption (see Valios 1997: 5). The BAAF study revealed, for example, that one out of every five black children adopted was, in fact, adopted by white people (see also the editorial 'Facts and fantasies', Community Care, 16–22 October 1997). None the less, in the latter half of 1998 it appeared that the Boateng was on something of a personal crusade to promote transracial adoption. Moreover, a good deal of his rhetoric appeared entirely at odds with the principles featured in the Children Act 1989 and social work policy and practice which had evolved in the 1980s and 1990s.

Throughout the last quarter of the twentieth century 'race' has featured as a key component in debates on adoption. In the early 1980s, in Britain, the Association of Black Social Workers and Allied Professionals (ABSWAP) challenged the hegemony of child placement policies and practices founded on a liberal and assimilationist perspective. The critique focused on the harmful consequences for black children of being placed with white adoptive and foster carers, but it, more broadly, drew attention to the impact of racism in British society (Small, 1982; Small with Prevatt Goldstein 2000). Associated with this critique were specific social work practice innovations, such as the influential New Black Families scheme, launched in the London Borough of Lambeth in 1980, which set out to recruit substitute black families for black children in the care of the local authority. Despite, as we saw in Chapter 2, a flawed approach to 'race' and ethnicity in the LAC system, a new attentiveness to such issues was gradually incorporated into practice guidelines for children in contact with social services and into the Children Act 1989. This legislation mandated that due consideration should be given to a child's 'race', language, religion and culture.

Specifically in terms of New Labour's ideas, developments in the United States may have played a part in terms of the 'inchoate backlash against a professional sensitivity to the "race" and ethnicity of children in need of placements' (Garrett 2000b; see also Garrett and Sinkkonen 2003). As argued earlier, this is particularly relevant given the cross-fertilisation of projects and strategies between Blair's New Labour and Clinton's Democrat administration (see also PIU 2000: 64). In the United States, following the passage of the Multiethnic Placement Act (MEPA) 1994 and the 1996 provisions on Removal of Barriers to Interethnic Adoption, it is now prohibited to use 'race' 'categorically or presumptively to delay or deny adoptive or foster care placements' (Brooks et al. 1999: 167). *Adoption: Achieving the Right Balance* (Department of Health 1998f), a circular issued in August 1998, stated that the 'Government has made it clear that it is unacceptable for a child to be denied loving adoptive parents solely on the grounds that the child and adopters do not share the same racial or cultural background' (Department of Health 1998f: para. 14). This perhaps reflected, therefore, not only New Labour's preoccupations, but – it might be suggested – aspects of the Clinton administration's child welfare agenda. Indeed, the connection between developments in relation to children and their families in the United States and in Britain will be returned to later in this chapter.

Significantly, however, *Adoption Now: Messages from Research* (Department of Health 1999b), an overview of recent adoption research published in October 1999, ran counter to New Labour's – at best – rather lukewarm support for same-'race' placements. The study concluded:

Whilst some white families can successfully parent children who are of a different ethnic origin from themselves, they have extra obstacles to surmount in ensuring that young people have a positive sense of themselves as members of a particular ethnic group. The requirement of the Children Act 1989 to seek to place children with parents who are of a similar cultural and ethnic background and who meet their needs provides a sound basis for policy. Placement with a family of a different ethnic and cultural background should be unusual and should be based on specific reasons for individual cases.

(Department of Health 1999b: 159)

Following the publication of the inquiry into the death of Stephen Lawrence and the fresh alertness to 'institutional racism', this was clearly a more restrained intervention on the question of 'race' and child placement than was apparent in some of the remarks of Boateng (Macpherson 1999). More measured, informed by research evidence and what was actually taking place in practice, *Adoption Now* cautioned against any radical departure from the principles of the Children Act 1989 and the dominant approach which had evolved and been implemented in the 1980s and 1990s. Although it will be argued in the next chapter that the DoH approach to such questions remains conceptually problematic, subsequent DoH reports on social services have since reinforced the importance, for children and their families, of 'race' and ethnicity (see Dutt and Phillips 2000; O'Neale 2000; SSI 2000a: ch. 6). The *Prime Minister's Review of Adoption* (PIU 2000) also failed to indicate any radical departures in terms of 'race' and the placement of children (see, however, Department of Health 2000e: 36).

More generally, Kirton (2000) has provided an authoritative overview of the main issues in relation to the same-'race' placement/transracial placement exchanges. A special issue of the journal *Adoption and Fostering* has similarly endeavoured to analyse the issue and to focus on complexities which have often been omitted in a debate which has been not only polemical (Gilroy 1994) but also reductionist because of the centrality of 'black' and 'white' dichotomies.

Blair takes control: remaking the social work approach to child adoption

This brief survey of developments and focal themes provides, therefore, part of the context for Blair's intervention on child adoption. At the launch of *Adoption Now*, in October 1999, the Health Minister, John Hutton, welcomed the 'record rise in the number of children being placed for adoption' in that 'for the first time in years' there had been a 'strong upward turn'. Figures revealed that adoptions had increased from 2,500 in 1997/8 to 2,900 in 1998/9, an increase of 16 per cent (Department of Health 1999c). The Minister also observed that New Labour's 'concerted campaign to place adoption at the forefront of options for children in care' was beginning to 'show results' and 'attitudes were finally changing' (Department of Health 1999c). The government circular of the previous year (Department of Health 1998f) and its associated publicity could, in part, have prompted this increase in the number of children adopted. Certainly local authorities appeared to be more intent on highlighting adoption, with Derbyshire County Council, for example, courting controversy by using the Internet to promote the adoption of children (see Valios 1999). However, in February 2000 it was announced that the Prime Minister was to personally chair a new Cabinet committee which was to radically review adoption law and procedures and to 'speed up' the adoption of 'looked after' children and young people who needed a permanent family. Crudely, in that it implied that a panacea was at hand, this announcement coincided with the publication of the Waterhouse report (2000) into the abuse of children in North Wales. It also followed Channel 4's screening of a series of programmes on child adoption which culminated in a bizarre 'trial' of Social Services Departments which were charged with failing 'looked after' children because of the dominant culture of 'political correctness' which continued to act as a brake on adoption.

In April 2000 the Social Services Inspectorate (SSI) issued its survey of local authority responses to *Adoption: Achieving the Right Balance* (SSI 2000a). In an accompanying letter, although conceding that many councils were performing 'very well', the Chief Inspector criticised the 'overall quality of adoption services' because they remained 'too variable to be acceptable'. One of the key findings, in the report, was that 2,400 children had been identified as suitable for adoption but had not been found families, while 1,297 adoptive families had been recruited and 'approved', but had not been found children to adopt (Department of Health 2000f). This prompted calls from Felicity Collier, chief executive of BAAF, for a national register of approved adopters who could be then viewed as a 'national resource', instead of the 'property' of individual local authorities which might not have the right children needing new families at a particular time (in Valios 2000a). This register idea was, moreover, one of the main agenda items at an extraordinary 'adoption summit' convened at Downing Street in late April (see Valios 2000b).

Reviewing the review

The *Prime Minister's Review of Adoption*, containing eighty-five recommendations, was published in July 2000. Criticising the overall 'lack of grip' in relation to child adoption, four key commitments centred on plans to: develop and implement a National Adoption Register; draw up new national standards which local authorities would be expected to follow; set up an 'Adoption and Permanency Taskforce' to promote best practice and tackle poor performance (see also Maluccio *et al.* 1986); and conduct a 'rapid scrutiny', or trawl, of the 'backlog' of children waiting to be placed with adoptive families and approved adopters waiting for children to see if any suitable matches could be made (PIU 2000: 4).

Throughout the late 1990s there was informed speculation that responsibility for adoption was to be taken away from local authorities and transferred to a new national organisation, or left entirely with voluntary adoption agencies (Welland 1999). However, the review recommended that adoption should remain a function of local authorities, although it was observed that 'significant improvements are sought in planning, decision-making, organisation and practice' (PIU 2000: 6). The idea of creating a central agency solely for recruiting adopters was also rejected (PIU 2000: 62). This task was to remain with local authorities, but consideration needed to be given to the setting of recruitment targets (PIU 2000: 65). It was also recommended that 'consideration should be given to allowing private companies to recruit, assess and prepare potential adopters' (PIU 2000: 58). Significantly, however, in response to the charge that social workers were hostile to child adoption, the review found 'little evidence of an institutional anti-adoption culture in social service departments' (PIU 2000: 26–7). In the context of allegations of 'political correctness' in the assessment of potential adopters, it was concluded that while 'there has been extensive media interest sparked by a relatively small number of instances, it is difficult to find consistent evidence about the degree to which unjustified discrimination applies' (PIU 2000: 41).

As will be suggested later there are a range of problems with the review and its implicit encompassing ideological framework, but it appeared, in general, to be a measured and restrained analysis of some of the key issues, particularly in the light of the political hyperbole attached to its initiation. It was also sensibly conceded that there was no 'magic bullet or simplistic quick fix' in relation to the problems identified (PIU 2000: 53). Perhaps on account of this note of appropriate caution, the review was criticised by the Conservatives and proponents of more radical 'reforms'. The shadow Health Secretary responded to the review by asserting that his party would not let the 'prejudices of a handful of politically correct bigots stand in the way of perfectly decent people being able to adopt children who need a secure and loving home' ('Ministers plan 50% increase in adoption', *The Guardian*, 8 July 2000). The director of the Adoption Forum argued that the document would serve only to 'shore up a seriously faulty edifice which leaves the architects of failure still in charge of the building' (in Winchester 2000a: 3).

In December 2000 the government published the White Paper *Adoption: a New Approach* (Department of Health 2000e). After the PIU report, it contained no unexpected or surprising departures. The aims of establishing a National Adoption Register and an Adoption and Permanency Task-force were presented once again. A new national target was to be set to increase the number of 'looked after' children adopted by 40 per cent by 2004/5. However, the aim, if possible, was to exceed this by achieving a 50 per cent increase. Other measures featured in the consultation paper included the plan to introduce new national standards for councils and adoption agencies. These were to be backed up with powers for 'emergency inspections' and 'special measures' to deal with wayward service providers. The White Paper also included the plan to introduce time scales which would result in a 'sound plan' being drawn up for the permanent future of a 'looked after' within six months of their starting to be continuously 'looked after'. Moreover, where the decision was made that adoption was the plan, a 'new family' should be found within a further six months. A new 'independent' review scheme was also envisaged for potential adopters whose application was rejected. In addition, new plans to support adoptive parents were briefly set out. Other key measures included: a new legislative option, termed 'special guardianship', which would provide permanence for a child but would fall short of the legal separation from birth parents involved in adoption; also identified was the plan to introduce a 'paramountcy' principle into adoption legislation (Department of Health 2000e; see also Ball 2001). In March 2001 a Bill was published, but it failed to be enacted before the general election in June. However, given the centrality of child adoption for New Labour it came as no surprise when the second Blair administration reactivated plans to legislate and the Adoption and Children Act received the royal assent in November 2002.

The rest of the chapter will now focus on specific criticisms of key elements in the New Labour approach to social work and child adoption. In addition, the aim will be to illuminate how the Prime Ministerial intervention connects with more embracing political preoccupations centred on, for example, the entitlement to Welfare services and parenting.

New Labour, old adoption

The high profile review and the subsequent White Paper risked creating the impression that there is an ample supply of children simply waiting to be 'rescued' from abusive children's homes. This implicit denigration of the 'looked after' system is paradoxical because New Labour has been intent on improving the 'quality' of care available for 'looked after' children and young people and has, as observed earlier, released additional financial resources under the QP programme (Department of Health 1998b; Secretary of State for Health 1998). As we have observed throughout Part II, problems remain with the New Labour approach to social work with children and families. However, unlike its Conservative predecessors, the Blair administration has not been content merely to 'warehouse' and vilify children in public care. None the less, there are risks that many parents – perhaps anxious that their children might be adopted – may be alienated and deterred from approaching local social services for 'family support'-orientated services. Related to this, the political centrality of child adoption could lead, of course, to the diminution of resources for such services (see also Department of Health, Department for Education and Employment, Home Office 2000).

Perhaps New Labour's presentation of child adoption also fails to adequately acknowledge that residential child care plays a vital role, for some children, within an integrated child welfare service. Less than 9 per cent of the 53,000 children in public care are, as the review conceded, in local authority community homes (PIU 2000: 10): the majority are in foster care and almost 75 per cent of the entire 'looked after' population of children, because of their legal status and location, are 'unlikely to require adoption' (Department of Health 1999b: 97). It is generally accepted that a high proportion of the remainder will be 'hard to place' for adoption (see, for example, 'Adopters shunning one in four children', *Community Care*, 7–13 November 2002: 7). Moreover, a recent study examining the perceptions of a small group of 'looked after' young people has revealed that many actually preferred residential homes to family-type placements (Berry 2001). Such findings are important if changes in the law on adoption are to meaningfully embrace, as the Children Act 1989 (section 1) at present directs, the 'ascertainable wishes and feelings of the child concerned'.

Significantly, a key expressed aim of the changes is to make the law more 'child-centred' and this was reflected in the intention to align adoption law with the Children Act 1989 and to ensure that a child's welfare is 'paramount'. However, the substance of this assertion has been somewhat undermined by New Labour's initial failure to consider the range of potential carers who may be available for a child. Despite moves in other jurisdictions to take account of more diverse family forms in adoption policy (Katz 2000), the government tried for months to reaffirm the existing position that only married couples or single people could adopt. None the less, as Ball (2001: 9) argued, if 'the principle that the child's welfare is "paramount" is to apply in relation to adoption, any restrictions which might otherwise deter suitable couples in a stable unmarried relationship from putting themselves forward as adopters appears contrary to that principle'. The New Labour position here did, however, sit more easily alongside the political aspiration of being 'entirely conventional' in terms of the attitude to the family. It was not until May 2002, after pressure from a coalition of nineteen agencies, that it was announced by the Health Secretary that MPs would be given a 'free vote' on an amendment to the Bill which would allow unmarried couples – which would include gays and lesbians – to jointly adopt.

Other criticisms that can be levelled at the government's approach are, perhaps, equally fundamental. The register, officially known as the Adoption and Children Act Register and administered by the Norwood Ravenswood charity, provides a 'national infrastructure for speeding up the process of matching' children in need of adoption with potential adopters and is a seemingly 'commonsense' response and practical innovation (PIU 2000: 57). However, implicit here is the notion that children awaiting adoption are mobile and – in the context of geographical supply and demand factors – can be removed from the environs of birth parents, friends and, if they are older, schools. These concerns have partly been addressed by the publication of a DoH circular, issued in August 2001, which mapped out how the register is likely to operate. However, the idea of a *national* matching scheme may still potentially run counter to other developments which take account of the 'openness' of adoption and post adoption 'contact' arrangements. It might also undermine a child's sense of continuity if there was an abrupt rupture caused by movement to another part of the country (see also Winchester 2000b). Importantly, unlike the PIU report, the White Paper stated that, subject to its age and level of understanding, a child's consent will need to be obtained before their name is featured on the register (Department of Health 2000e: 36). None the less, the register perhaps hints at the objectification of children who are 'looked after'. This interpretation is further substantiated by the jarring references, throughout the review, to the 'stock' of children in public care (see, for example, PIU 2000: 19, 86, 87).[1] This alienating and disparaging language, even redolent of Poor Law and workhouse discourses centred on the children of the poor and 'dangerous' classes, hardly evidences a 'new approach' which will be attentive and alert to the inevitably complex needs of *individual* children in need of permanent substitute care. It does, however, reflect aspects of New Labour's arid managerialism and the 'target'-setting orientation which seeks to 'modernise' the public sector and combat the 'forces of conservatism' (Department of Health 1998d: see also Hall 1993, 1998; Clarke and Newman 1997; Fawcett and Featherstone 1998; Powell 1999, 2000; Taylor-Gooby 2000).

Another criticism relates to birth families. As observed earlier, the register *could* lead to difficulties in terms of adoptees being able to maintain face-to-face contact with birth mothers and other relatives. More broadly, birth mothers – now more prominent in the discourse on adoption – continue to be dismissed and scornfully regarded by some of the proponents of more assertive and widespread adoption policies. For Morgan (1998: 7), for example, 'tormented birth mothers describing their regrets' have become 'along with sexual and reproductive peculiarities' the 'stock-in-trade of television talk shows'. In the early twenty-first century a certain cooling towards birth mothers is, perhaps, detectable in how research on adoption is at present marginalising these women. None of the studies featured in *Adoption Now*, for example, saw fit to have 'obtained the views of birth relatives' (Department of Health 1999b: 6). Indeed, partly mirroring these developments, there are some indications that New Labour longs for the old practices of child adoption, which pivoted on a definitive severance of the adopted child's relationship with its birth mother and family of birth. With this former approach to adoption, birth mothers were rendered entirely superfluous after the transfer of parental responsibility had taken place. The New Labour position is complex because there is a grudging recognition of birth mothers and other birth relatives. This is reflected in the new National Adoption Standards and, more specifically, in the new right birth relatives have to ask for an intermediary service so they can let an adopted adult know of their interest in making contact. However, undermining this is a more overriding and anachronistic perception of adoption as a 'one-off' event and not a lifelong process for all involved. This is apparent, for example, in the numerous references to adoption being a 'fresh start' for a child (Department of Health 2000e: 3, g). This psychologically crude and unconvincing idea of adoption as a 'fresh' or 'new' start for a child is, of course, deeply embedded in adoption discourse (see, for example, the debate on the Adoption of Children Bill 1926, *Hansard*, vol. 192, col. 926, February 1926). However, in a contemporary sense, birth mothers and birth relatives perhaps render the adoption of children unduly complex and introduce an untidy or messy component which is at odds with the managerialist orientation of New Labour. It is certainly clear, at the level of policy making, that there is a *new impatience* with birth families. We are advised, although no evidence is provided, that 'once a child has been admitted in LA [local authority] care the focus *too often* tends to be exclusively on rehabilitation with the birth family' (PIU 2000: 25, emphasis added). Similarly elsewhere, it is asserted that there is 'a perception that courts tend to give "the benefit of the doubt" to birth parents' (PIU 2000: 32). Furthermore, a SSI survey asserts that 'in resolving conflicts of interests there were situations when too much emphasis had been given to the wishes of birth families rather than the best interests of children' (SSI 2000c: 63–4).

In New Labour's discourse, this apparent aim of marginalising birth parents and birth families can also be perceived as bound up with the Blair administration's more general preoccupations and programmes concerned with social welfare provision and with families and parenting. As argued in Chapter 5, New Labour is heavily influenced by the 'Welfare reforms' of the former Clinton administration (see also, however, Pierson and Castles 2002). In this context, the US Adoption and Safe Families Act 1997 can be interpreted as reflecting a more directive and assertive approach to birth parents, since it 'places a strong emphasis on shortened timeframes for terminating parental rights and on adoption promotion' and undercuts the 'potential for strengthening family preservation services' (Kelly and Blythe 2000: 36; see also McGowan and Walsh 2000). Crudely put, if birth parents do not co-operate and meet certain behavioural requirements, they will 'lose' their children. Clearly, the New Labour plans are not as assertive, or drastic, as those of the Clinton administration, but the suggestion is that, albeit with significant differences, the government's approach can – once again – be situated on the same ideological terrain as the Democrats' approach to welfare and child adoption (see also Maza 2000; Katz 2000). The emergence of a new, 'tougher' approach to child adoption might be interpreted in this way as it relates to birth parents.[2]

Also important here is New Labour's apparent enthusiasm for recasting exclusionary classifications and typologies. This is reflected, as we saw in Chapter 5, in the re-emergence of so-called 'problem families', a construct, which comprised a focal part of social policy discourse in the 1950s (see Philp and Timms 1957; Hall 1960: ch. 10). Blair himself, when shadow Home Secretary, was apt to use the formulation (see *The Guardian*, 26 July 1993) and by the late 1990s the ideological category 'problem families' was being uncritically deployed, once again, in discourses centred on children and families (see Cleaver and Freeman 1995: 51–3; Department of Health 1995a; Eisenstadt 1998; Steele 1998). Indeed, in *imagining* and constructing some families in this way additional reasons are implicitly furnished for a potentially 'tougher' approach to child adoption and, more broadly, to child welfare as a whole.

In this context, perhaps the sad plight of Pat Amos illustrates the new 'tough' approach to wayward, recalcitrant and 'neglectful' mothers. A single parent with five children, she was sentenced to sixty days in Holloway prison, in May 2002, because two of her daughters had a poor school attendance record (see 'Truant mum is heroin addict', *Daily Mirror*, 20 May 2002). A columnist with *The Sun*, Jane Moore, summed up the vituperative tone of much of the media coverage of the family tragedy:

> It's an undeniable fact that imprisoning Pat Amos for the persistent truancy of her two daughters was an unmitigated success . . . It's the clearest sign yet that the government is finally getting to grips with stopping the rot of future generations bringing up children with the same disregard for authority. A suitably chastened Emma, 15, and Jackie, 13, dutifully traipsed off to their Banbury school safe in the knowledge that, if they didn't, mumsy would be back peeing in a bucket . . .

However – as is clear from this short extract – this New Labour morality tale, including its own 'what works' mini-narrative, contained many key themes and preoccupations which lie at the core of the Blairites' 'modernisation' project (see also 'Prison worked, says truants' mother', *The Guardian*, 27 May 2002).

Conclusion

The administrations of both Major and Blair have understood the potential of the emotive and popular appeal of a child adoption 'reform' agenda. In the words of the Prime Minister, the dominant approach is apt to be 'eye-catching' because adoption is situated at the intersection of a range of issues enmeshed in the social divisions and cleavages associated with social class, 'race' and ethnicity, sexual orientation, gender roles, age, (dis)ability. On account of this positioning it provides, therefore, a vehicle on which to transport a plethora of related political preoccupations and programmes. Put another way, adoption creates a wide discursive space for politics – particularly politics grounded in an 'entirely conventional' view of social relations. Related to this, of course, child adoption provides ample opportunity to caricature as a 'politically correct' fixation (occasionally simplistic) endeavours to redress discrimination and hardship.

The New Labour approach to child adoption can be understood partly as political opportunism. However, it also reflects a deeply rooted concern about reforming the 'looked after' system. Clearly, a number of more 'radical' reforms, such as removing the responsibility from local authorities, have been rejected. Blair's plans can, however, still be criticised for a tendency to objectify children in public care. This can be related to the government's managerialist orientation, and reservations have also been expressed, in this chapter, about the Adoption and Children Act Register and the implicit hankering for a return to anachronistic adoption policies and practices. In addition, the failure to properly appreciate the needs of birth mothers and other birth relatives can be viewed as reflective of New Labour's more encompassing ideological approach to Welfare services, the family and associated constructs of 'parenting'.

The more assertive approach to child adoption has also led to the suggestion that there is a 'danger of local authorities putting government adoption targets before the needs of individual looked after children' (Gupta 2002). More fundamentally, if child adoption must exist into the twenty-first century, then it must be radically different from that which evolved in Britain from the late 1920s. There can be no return to what Lowe (2000: 316) has termed the 'golden period of adoption' which stretched from 1951 to 1968 when there was greater availability of babies and adoption was conceived as a 'secret' event which radically ruptured a child's relationship with its birth family. Those who long for those days and for the social dynamics promoting this conceptualisation represent – to use the words of the Prime Minister – the 'forces of conservatism'.

This book is preoccupied with what we have termed the *remaking* of social work with children and families. However, one key aspect of social work, the dominant approach in relation to 'race' and ethnicity, has remained largely stable throughout the period under discussion. The next chapter will, therefore, critically focus on this aspect of theory and practice.

7

VIEWING THE WORLD THROUGH
A MONOCHROME LENS

Social work with children and families and the dominant approach to 'race' and ethnicity

Social work with children and families throughout the period covered in this book has been appropriately preoccupied with seeking to promote what has variously been described as 'anti-discriminatory practice' (Thompson 1997), 'anti-racist practice' (Dominelli 1988; Singh 1997; Williams 1999) and 'anti-oppressive practice' (Dalrymple and Burke 1995; Dominelli 1998; McDonald and Coleman 1999). These paradigms are historically rooted in the professional value base (Forsythe 1995), but also reflect more encompassing contemporary discourses which endeavour to engage with notions of 'diversity' and 'difference' (see also Williams *et al.* 1998; Garrett 2002). These ideas and aspirations to a better and fairer world are, as Naomi Klein (2000: ch. 5) has maintained, susceptible to transmutation by the forces of corporate capital (see also Alexander and Alleyne 2002: 542). None the less, within social work, much to the annoyance of social and political conservatives, recognition of diversity and difference must be addressed in education and training. In terms of practice, the Children Act 1989 also places a duty on local authorities to have regard to the 'religious persuasion, racial origin and cultural and linguistic background' of children in public care.

At the level of institutional practices, however, social work continues to fail to adequately respond to users of services who are black (Barn *et al.* 1997; Dutt and Phillips 2000; Parekh 2000).[1] More generally, the killing of Stephen Lawrence and the subsequent publication of the report of the Macpherson inquiry (1999) has highlighted the tenacity of anti-black racism and has, of course, directed attention to the 'institutional racism' embedded in the police and other sectors of the state (see also Lea 2000). The murder of Zahid Mubarek in Feltham Young Offenders' Institute (YOI) also points to the resilience of a type of racism, manifestly associated with fascist ideology, which is rooted in a potentially *lethal* antipathy to black people (Sivanandan 2000). The suggestion here, however, is that social work's approach to questions of 'race' and ethnicity, rooted in a more embedded discourse, has failed to address the specificity of Britain's *largest* ethnic minority, Irish people. Furthermore, an exploration of this Irish dimension provides us with a route into wider debates about 'race', ethnicity, migration and culture in contemporary Britain. Being prepared to re-examine this area is necessary because social workers will increasingly have to engage with dislocated and diasporic communities (Boyle 2001). The argument in this chapter, therefore, is that children's and families' social workers may be better able to respond to issues associated with 'race' and ethnicity if there is a new willingness to examine historical and contemporary responses to one of the oldest diasporic communities, the Irish community (see also Walter 2001: ch. 1).[2]

Initially, we will focus on social work's dominant approach to 'race' and ethnicity and the fixation with unitary and seemingly uncomplicated 'black' and 'white' categories. This will be followed by an analysis of social work's failure to meaningfully interrogate 'whiteness'. Next, the specificity of Irish people in Britain will be discussed. The focus will be on historical patterns of racialisation, exclusion and othering (see also Hickman 1998). It is then argued that any project centred on the remaking of social work with children and families in Britain needs to incorporate, at the level of theory and practice, an awareness of the contemporary specificity of Irish children and families. Equally important, social work needs to revitalise its critical interest in issues associated with 'race', ethnicity and (be)longing because of the contemporary trend in which DoH guidance and protocol documents are beginning to downgrade the importance of anti-discriminatory practice. A new attentiveness to this dimension of theory and practice is, moreover, important because of the contemporary treatment of refugees and asylum seekers.

Social work in a 'black' and 'white' world

It has been observed that – because of anti-racist endeavour – care plans, reviews and assessments are now, 'at least at procedural level . . . shot through with recognition of the service user's needs in terms of language, culture, religion, race and ethnicity; something that was not apparent ten years age' (Williams 1999: 219). However, this statement is highly debatable in terms of Irish children and families in Britain. A central factor has been the dominant conceptual paradigm which suggests that child-care issues associated with 'ethnic minorities' are meaningful solely in relation to children who are black (see O'Neale 2000). Clearly, these issues remain of vital importance to black children, but this reductive approach, with its 'monochrome lens', fails to respond adequately to many children with cultural needs arising from their specific national, or ethnic, background.

111

With social work, the 'misrecognition' of an Irish dimension to practice has tended to be institutionalised and has normally resulted in Irish people being encouraged to tick a 'white other' box on forms designed to monitor the 'race' and ethnicity of users of services (see also Fraser 2000: 115). Local authorities have also routinely failed to consult Irish people and Irish community groups when service plans are drawn up (Hickman and Walter 1997). Similarly, DoH policy documents which guide and direct social work practitioners and social work educators have routinely omitted Irish children from consideration when issues of 'race' and ethnicity are interrogated (see also, for example, Barn *et al.* 1997; Kirton 1999, 2000; Thoburn *et al.* 2000; Shepherd and Watkins 2000). In 2000, a number of years into the Blairite 'modernisation' drive, a report was published which purported to be an authoritative examination of services provided for 'ethnic minority children and families' (O'Neale 2000). Typifying the dominant approach, an accompanying press release asserted: '*Ethnic minority families face many issues that white members do not . . .*' (Department of Health 2000h, emphasis added). A short section of the report then set out how the term 'ethnic minority' was to be used: 'It specifically covers families from Africa, the Asian subcontinent, the Caribbean, British-born members of these groups and other people of mixed race, i.e. people with one black parent, *in other words people who are black*' (O'Neale 2000: 1, emphasis added).

Children who are Irish can, of course, also identify as black, yet essentially this DoH report failed, in truth, to provide a rounded overview of services for *all* ethnic minority children and families on account of the shrinking of 'race' and ethnic minority to a black/white binary. Given this approach, how, for example, could the DoH begin to form a view if services take account of the cultural and identity needs of, for example, a second-generation Irish boy being 'looked after' by English foster carers? Similarly, how might the department have perceived the services available for a girl from an Irish traveller family who has been placed in 'secure' accommodation because of criminal offences?[3] A more recent report from the DoH has called for all social services staff to 'become culturally competent', yet the continued promotion of a limited conceptual framework is likely to undermine this aspiration (SSI 2000c: 81). Furthermore, the dominant approach, with its casual disregard of the ethnicity of Irish children, would seem to run counter to the UN Convention on the Rights of the Child and the Human Rights Act 1998.

The *Framework for the Assessment of Children in Need and their Families*, as observed in Chapter 5, referred to 'inclusive practice' (Department of Health, Department for Education and Employment, Home Office 2000: 26–7). Strikingly, given the more familiar conceptual constraints, a section centred on 'inclusive practice' acknowledges:

> The population of England is comprised of many white minority ethnic groups as well as black minority ethnic groups and the differences in culture, religion, language and traditions for white minority groups have to be accounted for . . . There are also a number of white minority ethnic groups who experience oppression on the basis of their ethnic, cultural or religious identity. In assessing families these experiences should be acknowledged and addressed.
>
> (Dutt and Phillips 2000: 37)

Clearly, this statement is to be welcomed, since it explicitly begins to fracture the notion that 'white' people in Britain form an undifferentiated, homogeneous social category. The approach of Dutt and Phillips to 'white minority ethnic groups' also mirrors the more recent willingness to identify and respond to the heterogeneous nature of black experience(s) in Britain (see, for example, Modood *et al.* 1997; also Phoenix 1998). However, two problems continue to exist with this more 'inclusive' interpretative perspective. First, despite the critique featured in Parekh (2000), there is still unwillingness to *specifically* acknowledge Irish people in Britain. Second, it is asserted that whilst there 'are some similarities and parallels in the experiences of black and white minorities in Britain there is also fundamental difference. Institutional racism has resulted in the impairment of the life opportunities of black people in this country' (Dutt and Phillips 2000: 37). This statement is accurate, yet there needs to be some qualification. Clearly, black people in Britain are subject to 'institutional racism', but Dutt and Phillips risk obscuring the fact that Irish people in Britain are *also* subject to racism (Hickman and Walter 1997; Parekh 2000: 61; see also 'Victory in racial abuse battle', *The Irish Post*, 17 February 2001) In the context of the research literature available, there is also an inexcusable failure to even begin to explore the situation of Irish children and families in Britain. This omission is, moreover, connected with a pervasive reluctance to begin to interrogate and deconstruct 'whiteness' in Britain. None the less, it is this 'whiteness' which is the absent centre around which the mainstream social work discourse on 'race' and ethnicity continues to circulate.

Social work and the 'empty' white category

In February 2000 the Department of Health conducted the first comprehensive survey of all 'children in need' in England. Undertaken under the QP initiative, this survey was also significant in that local authorities were asked to classify children according to the ethnic categories used in the subsequent 2001 census (http://www.doh.gov.uk/cin/cin2000results.htm).

This survey found that 16 per cent (37,500) of 'children in need' were 'minority ethnic' children and 82 per cent were 'white'.[4] This approach again suggests that Irish children – *likely* to be white – are not a 'minority ethnic' group. However, because this survey deployed the categories used in the 2001 census, the DoH was also able to provide information on 'white Irish' children. Estimates indicated that 1 per cent (1,700) of 'children in need' in England fell into this category; 600 of these children were 'looked after' and 1,100 were 'supported in their families or independently'. A similar DoH survey, conducted in September/October 2001, revealed that there were 1,600 'white' Irish children in need in England (www.doh.gov.uk/cin/cin2001results.htm). These figures are problematic for a number of reasons and they are likely to underestimate the number of 'children in need' who are likely to self-identify as Irish. It is also significant that one of the tables provided in this exercise – specifically table 10 in both surveys – again seeks to situate Irish children *outside* ethnic status and *inside* a homogenised 'white' category.

Despite the rather ambiguous changes reflected in these surveys, social work's response to questions of 'race' and ethnicity remains underpinned by a perception of 'whiteness' as a universally dominant, homogeneous and static social category (see Bonnett 2000). Whiteness 'certainly carries privileges, but they are not always guaranteed', and in order to 'give back meaning to the apparent emptiness of the "white" category it is necessary to explore the specificity of white experiences' (Walter 2001: 6; see also Brah 1992; Maynard 1994). Clearly, in terms of historical and contemporary processes of racialisation, 'whiteness' has been 'enormously, often terrifyingly effective in unifying disparate groups of people' (Dyer 1997: 19). None the less, 'some are more securely white than others' and this is reflected in the creation of people who are 'sometimes whites' (Dyer 1997: 4). That is to say, some – such as Irish people or Jewish people – may be 'let into whiteness under particular historical circumstances' (Dyer 1997: 19). In short, 'whiteness' as a category is socially constructed and contains a shifting border and internal hierarchies. In the context of the current discussion, the construction of Irish people has, of course, been inseparable from factors connected with British colonialism and the temper of Anglo-Irish relations at particular moments in history (see Busteed 1999: 103).

Perhaps social work also needs to recognise that the centrality of the black/white binary is related to the fallacious idea that, until the 1950s, Britain was a 'homogeneous white country' (Alibhai-Brown 2000: 29). Integral to this myth of homogeneity was the implicit assertion that all people 'who were white assimilated into the "British way of life" and that the problems all resided with those who migrated and possessed a different colour of skin' (Hickman 1998: 299). This idea also helped to mask the 'internal ethnic, regional and national differences which characterise the "United Kingdom"' (Hickman 1998: 290; see also Parekh 2000: 61).

Moreover, it also served to bind together, within a gradually diminishing empire, internal forces with materially opposed class interests.

Related to 'whiteness' and the British 'national story', the denial of the specificity of the cultural and national background of Irish children in Britain, can, in an historical sense, be linked with social construction of the 'British childhood' and this was reflected in the discursive practices of the welfare state from the nineteenth century until, perhaps, the late 1960s (see Hendrick 1990). Education played a key role, both in terms of state provision and – for Irish children – the schooling provided by the Roman Catholic Church in Britain. Not all Irish children are, of course, Roman Catholics, but historically, for Hickman (1996), the Roman Catholic Church in Britain can be perceived as seeking to 'incorporate and denationalise' Irish people with Roman Catholic schools, particularly, holding up 'a mirror to their pupils in which was reflected their Catholicity rather than their Irishness'. (See also, however, the report of the Working Party on Catholic Education in a Multiracial, Multicultural Society 1984.) This approach had similar consequences in relation to the intervention of Catholic child welfare and 'rescue' organisations in Britain in that the Catholicism of potential adopters was the prime factor in relation to, for example, the adoptive placement of Irish children. Furthermore, partly because of the absence of legal adoption until 1952 in the Republic of Ireland, the Roman Catholic Church there operated as something of a transmission belt for 'illegitimate' children: helping, in fact, to organise their dispersal within, but also from, Ireland to childless Roman Catholic couples in, for example, the United States (Newman 1951; see also Roth 1980; Milotte 1997). Indeed, English Catholics adopted many Irish children, particularly in the 1950s and 1960s, but their Irish – national and wider cultural heritage was apt to be lost to them (see Milotte 1997). These Irish children, whilst retaining their Catholic heritage, were subjected to processes of 'incorporation' and 'denationalisation' and this has had consequences for some of the adoptees who now feel that their concept of self and sense of identity have been undermined (Hosegood 1993; Palme 1999).

'Problem families' and the racialisation of Irish children and families

In the 1950s many families of the urban poor were characterised as 'problem families' who were indolent, feckless, dirty and a drain on the resources of the post-war welfare state (see Philp and Timms 1957; Hall 1960: ch. 10; Starkey 2000). Welshman (1999) has explored how social work in Britain related to 'problem families' and, as we saw towards the end of the previous chapter, this construct has emerged, once again, in social work and social care discourses. However, in the context of the theme at the core of this chapter, 'problem families' can also be interpreted as part of a matrix of ideas historically preoccupied with Irish people in Britain. In the early 1950s, for example, Spinley (1953) provided an account of 'one of the worst slums in London'. She went on to describe a district which was 'notorious . . . for vice and delinquency . . . a major prostitution area' and the 'blackest spot in the city for juvenile delinquency'. In this area, she asserted 'a large proportion of the inhabitants are Irish; social workers say: "The Irish land here, and while the respectable soon move away, the ignorant and the shiftless stay"' (Spinley 1953: 40). The author, possessing the 'stigmatising gaze of a culturally dominant other' (Fraser 2000: 109), then sought to provide her readers with a picture of a typical house in the locality:

> The most noticeable characteristic of the house is the smell, indeed on a first visit the middle-class stomach may find it impossible to stay longer than five minutes. These strong odours are partly due to the fact windows are not opened and so no current of air can carry away the smells of cooking, lavatory bucket, mattress wet in the night, and the baby's vomit hurriedly wiped up.
>
> (Spinley 1953: 40)

Descriptions such as this are recursive in that similar representations of the living conditions of Irish people were produced in the nineteenth century (see, for example, Engels 1926). Such accounts are also reflective of more embedded and pervasive processes of 'othering' in that the experience of Irish people in Britain has been framed by the 'construction of the Irish (Catholic) as a historically significant Other of the English/British (Protestant)' (Hickman 1998: 290–1; see also Gilley 1999). In this context the identification of 'dirt' and 'dirtiness' has, moreover, fulfilled a significant function. Indeed, it is often the case that racist discourses have associated black people 'in various ways with dirt . . . notably in the repeated perceptions' that they smell or their food smells (see Dyer 1997: 75–6). As Spinley's account clearly highlights, similar linkages have been made in relation to Irish people in debates, within social work and social policy, on the 'problem family'.

More broadly, Delaney (1999) has examined the responses of the British state to Irish immigration during the period stretching from Ireland's semi-independence in the early 1920s until the end of the Second World War. He found that the issue of deportation – more specifically British ruminations on the viability of *enforcing* deportation – featured as a recurring subtext in Anglo-Irish relations during the late 1920s and 1930s (see also, in this context, Garrett 2003a). In 1937, for example, an inquiry was even held, in the House of Commons, to ascertain whether it would be 'possible to put an import duty on Southern Irish human beings as it is placed on

Southern Irish animals?' (*Hansard*, 321, col. 147, March 1937). In the 1940s also there were suggestions that 'the flow of people from Eire' could be 'diverted to the Dominions' (see Walshaw 1941: 77). Irish people from the southern state were granted a privileged position, in relation to those from other countries, under the British Nationality Act 1948. Irish citizens were also exempted from the provisions of the Commonwealth Immigrants Act 1962 (see Miles 1993), but these exemptions largely related to complications caused by the partitioning of Ireland and continuing labour shortages in Britain after the Second World War. However, Irish exclusion from the tightening up of the immigration process should not necessarily be interpreted as representing tolerance and acceptance of Irish people. The Commonwealth Immigrants Bill had, in fact, made Irish people subject to immigration control and some British MPs were of the opinion that Irish immigrants might undermine and contaminate Britain. One MP, reflecting some of the same themes featured in Spinley's account, stated that Irish people, on account of tuberculosis, were 'far more likely to cause danger of infection to other people' than were Commonwealth immigrants. He also proposed that Irish people should be able to remain in Britain for 'a certain period only' (*Hansard*, cols 753–7, 6 November 1961; see also the comments of Denis Healey MP in Hickman 1998: 302).

Recognising Irish specificity

Returning to the present day, transformations have clearly taken place in the perception of Ireland and 'Irishness' and these are likely to impact on social work perceptions. In the late 1990s and early twenty-first century, politicians and commentators, for example, have looked on, in puzzled wonderment, at the arrival of the so-called 'Celtic tiger' economy in the Republic of Ireland (see Kirkby *et al.* 2002). Indeed, one national British newspaper has asserted that the Irish, with their allegedly ostentatious new-found wealth, are the 'playboys of Europe' (*The Observer*, 22 July 2001). Representations of Irish people have also tended to centre on popular culture: the *Riverdance* phenomenon, U2 and the Corrs, the boom in fake Irish pubs (Stevens *et al.* 2000; see also West 2002). Indeed, the popularity of a particular construction of Irishness led one British newspaper to contend, in the mid-1990s, 'If you're hip, you must be Irish' (O'Sullivan 1996). In the same article one writer and cultural commentator mused: 'Irish culture is seductive. It has become a signifier for hedonism with soul.' More generally, within the field of cultural studies, it has been claimed that 'Irishness' has 'cachet' and that it has attained the 'status of cultural capital' (Thompson 2001: 1; see also, however, Maddox 1996).

With social work in Britain, however, there is still an embedded failure to recognise the specificity of the *actual* experience(s) of Irish children and families. Related to this, it should be acknowledged that being Irish in

117

Britain can also be associated with a number of interconnected, far from 'hip', hardships. Indeed, a major study published by the Commission for Racial Equality (CRE) indicates that, in the early twenty-first century, some understanding of a number of key factors should inform social work assessments and, more broadly, aspects of service planning in relation to Irish children in Britain (see Hickman and Walter 1997). Important factors relate to racism, health, labour and housing market locations, and policing.

Irish children and families in Britain are still subject to racism (Engels 1926; Walter 1995; Hickman and Walter 1997; Parekh 2000; Walter 2000; see also 'Irish Centre suffers third strike by racist vandals', *The Irish Post*, 18 May 2002). This racism is, moreover, embedded in scientific discourse (Eysenck 1971) and popular culture. Importantly, both Ullah (1985) and Walter and Hickman (1997) have also found widespread anti-Irish prejudice amongst schoolchildren in Britain. The CRE report, for example, found that harassment of second-generation Irish children in schools was reported by 22 per cent of their sample.

As suggested earlier, anti-Irish racism is apt to be masked by a superficial fixation with Irish popular culture, or admiration for the performance of the economy in the southern state. However, even within contemporary liberal discourse a contemptuous attitude to Irish people often resurfaces. A popular national newspaper columnist has, for example, contrasted Ireland's 'renaissance' with 'the old pre-boom Ireland of hopeless old piss-heads doing zilch' (*The Observer Magazine*, 11 March 2001; see also Burchill 2002). Furthermore, an interchange of anti-Irish and anti-black discourses can be seen to have operated at various tiers within the state in Britain and these have been different, but often discursively enmeshed (see also Brah 1992; in Hickman 2000: 52). The notion of 'swamping', reactivated by Home Secretary David Blunkett, illuminates this fluidity. The idea of a black presence 'swamping' Britain was, of course, used in the 1980s by the Prime Minister, Margaret Thatcher (see Scraton 1987). However, the previous decade, a key social work textbook had similarly observed that 'fears have sometimes been expressed' that Irish immigrants will 'swamp the social services with their demands' (Cheetham 1972: 18; see also Walter 2001: 91).

The stress prompted by anti-Irish racism is, perhaps, also related to the relatively poor health of Irish people in Britain (see Tilki 1998; Bracken and O'Sullivan 2001). Indeed, Irish men are the *only* migrant group whose mortality is higher in Britain than in their country of origin (Hickman and Walter 1997; see also Greenslade 1992; Tilki 1998; Parekh 2000: 178; Harding and Balarajan 2001). Second-generation Irish people in Britain are also less healthy than the general population (Pearson *et al.* 1991; Campbell 1999). Moreover, the rates of admission to hospital for Irish people are higher than those of a number of other groups, so also is the incidence of schizophrenia (Greenslade 1992). The health of the Irish in

Britain is also likely to be related to the labour market and housing sector location. This is also distinct and should be addressed in social services' strategic planning and in social work and wider social welfare engagements with individual Irish children (Hickman and Walter 1997).

On account of the operation of the Prevention of Terrorism Acts (Hillyard 1993), Irish people have been subjected to differential policing and this continues despite the 'peace process' (see, for example, 'Police watch ferry passengers', *The Irish Post*, 28 October 2000; also 'Protests over plans to treat Irish as suspects', *The Irish Times*, 11 December 2000). In addition, other parts of the criminal justice system appear to relate to Irish people in a discriminatory way (Mooney and Young 1999; see also 'Irish suicides spark claims of vendetta in British prison', *The Observer*, 27 October 2002). In summary, contemporary research findings in these areas would not seem to support the 'ethnic fade' thesis which assumes that Irish people have been   and continue to be   rapidly assimilated and so are 'just the same' as 'white' British people in terms of life chances and interactions with state institutions.

Since 1995 the CRE has recognised that Irish people are a distinct ethnic group. In terms of social work's institutional practices, as observed earlier, the Framework has tried to promote the idea of 'inclusive practice' and associated 'race' and ethnic monitoring materials also include a new '*white* Irish' category. Despite problems with this category and the encompassing approach, the Framework could still provide a lens through which the social and cultural needs of Irish children could be recognised. In addition, the Human Rights Act 1998 may form part of the legal backdrop for promoting changes in social work theory and practice. The United Convention on the Rights of the Child also suggests that the specificity of the cultural needs of Irish children should be taken more seriously by social workers and other social care professionals. Article 8, for example, calls on states to 'respect the right of the child to preserve his or her identity' including 'nationality'. Similarly, the substitute care of children calls for 'due regard' to be paid to the 'desirability of continuity in a child's ethnic, religious, cultural and linguistic background'.

Social theory and welfare practices need, therefore, to evolve in order to take account of the historical and contemporary specificity of Irish children and families in Britain. However, this is not to suggest that Irish people form a homogeneous and socially static bloc (see Hall 1992; Hobsbawm 1996; Fraser 2000; Parekh 2000; Lentin 2001). This chapter is not, moreover, seeking to promote a crude essentialism or dangerous 'ethno-dogma' (Gilroy 1994; see also Brah 1992). As Gilroy (1994) counsels, we should be wary of reifying 'race' and ethnicity so that they appear as *things* rather than *processes.* This understanding remains crucial when, as Brah (1992: 43) suggests, 'social phenomena such as racism seek to fix and naturalise difference and create impervious boundaries between groups'.

Furthermore, as argued elsewhere, 'like other communities, the Irish community is complex and diverse – potentially energised, in fact, as much by difference and hybridity as by a sense of commonality' (Garrett 1998: 38; see also Anthias and Yuval-Davis 1993: ch. 6). Similarly processes of racialisation and 'othering' cannot be detached from social divisions rooted in social class and gender (see also Edge 1995; Walter 1995; Hickman and Walter 1997; Maguire 1997; Kanya-Forster 1999; Gray 2000; Walter 2001; see also Marston 2002). In addition, there are specific factors attached to the age and generation of Irish people in Britain (Ullah 1985; Campbell 1999; see also Norman 1985). Religion and religious affiliation have, of course, also been a significant factor (Gilley 1999; Pooley 1999). This is not, however, to suggest that anti-Irish racism has been directed only at Roman Catholic migrants from Ireland (Hickman and Walter 1997; see also Walter 2001: 164–5).

Arguably, alterations of systems relating to the monitoring of 'race' and ethnicity, prompted in part by changes introduced in the 2001 census, seem to be beginning to produce better recording of Irish ethnicity and this may begin, over time, to impact on social work practice with children and families.[5] This is clearly important and runs counter to the wishes of those – often on the political right – with a deep antipathy to this form of monitoring (see, in this context, Williams 2002). The Parekh report – *The Future of Multi-ethnic Britain* – whilst stressing that people have 'multiple identities', has also endeavoured to highlight the specificity of Irish people in Britain (Parekh 2000: 10). It acknowledges, for example, that 'around 3 million Irish people in Britain are by far the largest migrant community'. However, 'all too often they are neglected in considerations of race and cultural diversity . . . It is essential . . . that all such considerations should take their perceptions into account' (Parekh 2000: 31). It is, however, conceded that some of the issues at the heart of this chapter are highly complex. For example, how individual Social Services Departments address the 'identity' aspects of children they 'look after' is vital. Yet this area should not be approached in a crude or simplistic manner, nor should responses pivot on stereotypical, constraining or anachronistic constructs of 'Irishness'. More prosaically, but just as important, it is the willingness of Social Services Departments to bolster what can, on occasion, be perceived as a fairly abstract commitment to provide culturally appropriate services with the funding of specific initiatives which will practically address the issue.

'Race', ethnicity, asylum seekers and refugees

A new willingness to question dominant approaches to 'race' and ethnicity is, moreover, vital in the context of increasing population movements across national boundaries. This is because mainstream discourse on 'race' and ethnicity is also apt to fail to take account of other ethnicities – other than Irish – not located in a 'black' category (see also Roskill 2000; Smith 2000). For example, the dominant theoretical understanding risks failing to adequately conceptualise the situation of many recent child migrants seeking refuge and asylum in Britain (see Cohen 1994; Williams *et al.* 1998; Castles and Davidson 2000; Parker 2000). In 2001 alone, for example, 2,735 unaccompanied children applied for asylum (ADSS 2002a: 4). Equally worrying, the dominant approach can be interpreted as providing political opportunists with the conceptual space to assert that punitive policies directed at refugees and asylum seekers are *not* racist because some of the people in these categories cannot be identified as 'black' (Yuval-Davis 2001). So, for example, the Race (Amendment) Act 2000 draws public bodies into the remit of legislation for the first time, yet the government outlaws only *colour* discrimination in the immigration service, 'leaving immigration officers free to discriminate against Tamils, Kurds, Roma and Afghans at will at the point of entry' (Back *et al.* 2002: 452; see also Cohen 2002; Sales 2002).

More broadly, as Arun Kundnani (2001: 43) has observed:

> In Britain, at precisely the time the Macpherson report into the murder of Stephen Lawrence was meant to usher in an anti-racist consensus across society, the asylum seeker issue has been an open wound through which racism has reinfected the body politic, combining with and reinforcing other forms of racism. [See also Parekh 2000: 212–17.]

In political terms this was evident, of course, in the speech of the then Conservative Party leader, William Hague, when in March 2001, he evoked an image of Britain becoming a 'foreign land' with its Anglo-Saxon heritage and character eroded (see Alexander and Alleyne 2002: 542). Partly mirroring developments elsewhere in Europe, there has also been a resurgence of far right activity with the British National Party (BNP) even managing to win a handful of council seats. As observed earlier, remarks from New Labour government Ministers have failed to respond adequately and may have contributed to the growth of racism. This has, of course, been evidenced by New Labour's response to asylum seekers and refugees and, as noted earlier, in the Home Secretary's unapologetic references to 'swamping' (see 'Blunkett defends "swamping" remark', *The Guardian*, 25 April 2002; 'Blunkett deeper in "swamp" row', *The Guardian*, 26 April 2002; see also 'Anger at new advice to Asians', *The Guardian*, 16 September 2002). In terms of legislation, the so-called Terrorism Act 2000 has also led to a widening sense of stigma for many refugee communities (see also 'Home Office films Roma deportation', *The Guardian*, 21 September 2002). The processes which result in the vilification and exclusion of asylum seekers and refugees are underpinned by a 'vicious circle logic of suspicion and deterrence' (Kundnani 2001: 42). Furthermore, such processes run entirely counter to ideas about 'inclusive practice' which are, at least rhetorically, central to the remaking of social work with children and families (Department of Health, Department for Education and Employment, Home Office 2000: 26–7).

Clearly, issues bound up with exclusionary practices directed at Irish people and asylum seekers from places as diverse as, for example, Iraq, Turkey, Romania and Kosovo are not the same. However, the key point here has been that 'binarized ways of thinking' (Jackson 1998: 104) and essentialist categories, such as 'black' and 'white', fail to provide the conceptual space from which to even begin to adequately address how groups and individuals are discriminated against (see also Pilkington 2003). Importantly, how asylum seekers are theoretically regarded is not, moreover, a mere abstract consideration: it is now central to contemporary social work practice with children and families. The survey carried out in September/October 2001, referred to earlier, indicated that some 6 per cent (12,600) of 'children in need' in England are now asylum-seeking children (www.doh.gov.uk/cin/cin2001results.htm). The providers of social work and social care are, as we saw in Chapter 2, also becoming more and more involved in 'scrutinising immigration status' (Sales 2002: 461). As Steve Cohen (2002: 538) has asserted:

> What is remarkable about modern immigration controls is the all-powerful position of the Home Office over all other government bodies. This is 'joined up' government with a vengeance. The Home Office does not operate simply as one department among several; rather, the entire state machinery – and particularly its agencies of welfare – are being co-opted into immigration enforcement, and this machinery is being orchestrated by, and is ultimately answerable to, the Home Office. In the relationship of power within the state, it is clear the Home Office quite consciously has its own 'big plan', and the plan is to transform the public and private sectors and the local state into agents of control.

Conclusion

The more socially progressive currents within social work need, therefore, to be alert to this new policing role. Equally important, as argued throughout this chapter, is the need to evolve more complex ways of understanding 'race', ethnicity and xeno-racism. Given that, organisationally, social work with children and families is in flux, it may, however, be a propitious moment to destabilise embedded approaches to these questions. In the next chapter, therefore, we will shift the focus and explore some of these organisational changes and look at how social work with children and families is now, in the new welfare domains of the Third Way, having to engage with a plethora of 'emergent professionals'.

8

SOCIAL WORK WITH CHILDREN AND FAMILIES IN A WORLD OF 'EMERGENT NEW PROFESSIONALS'

The Connexions Service (CS), also simply described as Connexions, is to provide a universal service dispensing information, advice and guidance to all thirteen to nineteen-year-olds.[1] Consultation relating to the new scheme took place in autumn 1999 and was followed by the setting up of a number of 'pathfinder', or pilot, projects. From April 2001 the Connexions Service, as a whole, began to be phased in and this is likely to continue for two or three years until it becomes fully operational (DfEE 2000a: 33). Some social workers may, for example, have the opportunity to become a personal adviser (PA). Others, if not wanting to become one of these 'emergent new professionals', are still likely to encounter a personal adviser and the Connexions Service in their daily work with children and families (DfEE 2000b: 7). Aspects of the thinking, in relation to youth support, underpinning the new initiative also gel with the Children (Leaving Care) Act 2000. The Connexions Service will, moreover, form a key component of the 'joined up' approach to the delivery of Welfare and education services by building on 'the best of multi-agency working' (DfEE 2000a: 56).

The chapter will begin by highlighting key aspects of Connexions and its overarching strategy. The first part will, therefore, be largely descriptive and will synthesise some of the main features of the Connexions Service and the personal adviser as articulated in a range of official sources (DfEE 2000a, b, c). The next section will examine, in more detail, how the Connexions Service and personal advisers may impact on social workers and local authority Social Services Departments. This will pay particular attention to the approach taken to engaging with young people. The Connexions Service and the personal adviser will also be situated in relation to more encompassing social and political preoccupations connected with youth transitions, social exclusion and disaffection, risk and the surveillance of young people. The concluding part of the chapter will then ponder on the possible impact of the growth of the personal advisers and mentors on social work recruitment.

Dealing with the 'drop-out' generation

Connexions has been viewed as 'the muscle behind Labour's rhetorical assault on the drop out generation' (Prasad 2001). Part of the basis for the Connexions Service was research which discovered that the proportion of sixteen to eighteen-year-olds not in education, training or work was as high as 9 per cent (DfEE 2000a: 14; see also DfEE 1999; Social Exclusion Unit 1999). However, Britain, of course, is not alone in its concern about young people's failure to engage with the 'world of work' and with educational services which facilitate the entry of young workers into the labour market. Thus the discourse centred on the Connexions Service refers to developments elsewhere. We have seen throughout the latter half of the book that New Labour is apt to be influenced by social policy 'innovations' in the United States and a number of references are made to the Gear Up youth programme which operates there (DfEE 2000a; see also Mead 1997; Deacon and Mann 1999; McGregor 1999; Walker 1999; Deacon 2000; Handler 2000; Swanson 2000; Prideaux 2001). However, schemes which resemble the fledgling Connexions Service are also identified in France and the Nordic countries of Norway and Denmark (DfEE 2000a: 28–30; see also Higham 2001).

The Connexions Service will, we are told, make available 'the best possible support in the transition from adolescence to adulthood' (Blair 2000: 4). In addition, the agency will create 'a radical new approach' which will 'overcome the fragmentation of much of current services' (DfEE 2000a: 9). At present it is still rather unclear how the agency will practically function, but at its core will be a network of personal advisers. The agency is also committed to the 'eight key Connexions principles' focused on: raising aspiration; meeting individual needs; taking account of the views of young people; inclusion; partnership; community involvement and neighbourhood renewal; extending opportunity and equality of opportunity; evidence-based practice (DfEE 2000b: 15).

Significantly, especially given the privatisation of the Careers Service, the Connexions Service will be a 'modern *public service*', yet it will be 'modern' in the New Labour sense of the term (DfEE 2000a: 5, emphasis added). In short, it will be an 'outcome-driven service' (DfEE 2000a: 34), armed with a 'range of cross-cutting targets' (DfEE 2000c: 11) and aspiring to 'excellence' (DfEE 2000c: 29). A cross-departmental CS national unit, based in Sheffield and London, has overall responsibility for the service (Weinstock 2000). However, it will enter into contract arrangements with locally based Connexions partnerships for the delivery of services. The national unit will, though, retain responsibility for the monitoring performance (DfEE 2000a: ch. 6; see also Fawcett and Featherstone 1998).

The 'emergent new professional': the personal adviser

At the 'heart of the service', therefore, is the personal adviser (DfEE 2000b: 7). This 'emergent professional' will be responsible for a range of work which will cut across the activity of other professionals, such as local authority child and family social workers. This is illustrated, for example, in the description of some of the activities of the personal adviser referred to as 'Pam' in the Connexions pamphlet *Get involved . . . make a difference*. More generally, the personal adviser will, we are advised:

> for the first time offer a single accountable professional to provide one-to-one support for young people and to oversee the effectiveness of interventions. They will be equipped with the knowledge and skills to provide information, advice and guidance on education/career pathways, health, social welfare and justice issues as well as the knowledge when to refer young people to a specialist service.
>
> (DfEE 2001c: 5)

In a speech to the Institute of Career Guidance, Anne Weinstock, the head of the Connexions Service, compared the role of the personal adviser to 'that of the triage nurse who assesses and arranges treatment in order of urgency' (Weinstock 2000). The personal adviser will, moreover, be 'drawn from a range of backgrounds and will be 'representative of the population' (DfEE 2000b: 8). The literature focused on the creation of the personal adviser also locates the arrival of this 'emergent professional' alongside related developments which point to the, more general, growth in mentors and advisers (see also, in this context, Donzelot 1979). This includes learning mentors within schools, the young persons' adviser for care leavers and New Deal personal advisers within the Employment Service (DfEE 2000b: 7; see also Ministerial Group on the Family 1999; Jordan 2000).

The personal adviser for most thirteen to sixteen-year-olds will be the learning mentor based in school. Similarly, the care leaver personal adviser, introduced under the Children (Leaving Care) Act 2000 for young people in public care, will act as the CS adviser for this group of young people (see also Calder 2000). Otherwise, personal advisers will maintain a 'shopfront presence' and will be deployed in a variety of locations, including schools, FE colleges and community settings. In terms of the daily operational management of personal advisers there will be a 'supervisory model akin to youth work and social work, that is, with a team leader' (DfEE 2000b: 16).

Further emphasising the spread of what Jordan (2000: 70) has referred to as 'tutelary bureaucracy', personal advisers will also operate with groups of 'mentors' drawn 'from local communities' who will have an important job to fulfil in 'providing role models and encouragement' for some young people (DfEE 2000a: 44). Policy guidance suggests that the Connexions Service 'will be responsible for drawing together a pool of mentors, perhaps by subcontract, managing the caseloads and working with them to develop their expertise in supporting young people' (DfEE 2000a: 44). Becoming a mentor could also become a first step on the ladder to becoming a fully fledged personal adviser (DfEE 2000a: 44).

Perhaps unsurprisingly, given New Labour's enthusiasm for public/private partnerships, employers will 'play an important role in the Connexions Service' and will be encouraged to provide mentors (DfEE 2000a: 44; see also Sivanandan 1998/9). This in the context of employers 'becoming increasingly involved in education locally' (DfEE 2000a: 44). However, employer involvement touches on the issue of young people's ability to choose their own personal adviser. They might not, for example, want one of the people responsible for monitoring their performance at work and for paying their salary providing 'advice' and 'guidance' on matters unrelated to their place of work. It is conceded that the young people consulted were in agreement that 'young people themselves should be involved in' either 'deciding' or 'having a say in who a personal adviser should be' (DfEE 2000a: 56), yet it is unclear what mechanisms are in place to ensure that this actually occurs. There also remains, of course, a good deal of ambiguity in the preceding sentence in terms of the ability of young people to meaningfully contribute to the process.

Personal advisers will work with schools, colleges and training providers. Their chief role, however, will be providing one-to-one support, information, advice and guidance to young people. They must, therefore, 'have the skills to assist the young person in navigating key life episodes' (DfEE 2000b: 8). Importantly, personal advisers will also be responsible for the 'assessment, planning and review' of young people. They will also endeavour to work with parents and carers and will be intent on 'encouraging high expectations in the home setting' (DfEE 2000b: 10). More generally, it will be the aspiration of personal advisers to 'contribute to neighbourhood renewal by ensuring that all sectors of the community are consulted and involved in the education and development of young people' (DfEE 2000a: 10). Personal advisers will work with other agencies, but also pay particular attention to keeping in contact with and monitoring their 'caseloads'. To aid this process the Connexions Service will have a 'reliable database of all 13–19 year-olds'. This database, to be discussed in more detail later in the chapter, will be a 'means to monitor the progress and outcomes of those individuals receiving in-depth or specialist support and those in target groups' for the Connexions Service (DfEE 2000b: 11; see also DfEE 2000a: 57). Personal advisers will, we are assured, also be subject to 'stringent vetting procedures' in the context of child protection (DfEE 2000b: 11).

A training framework is being established to enable personal advisers to meet and deliver key functions of their role (DfEE 2000a: 12). This training will 'take account of and develop' four 'skills and knowledge areas': information gathering and assessment; planning, intervention, support and guidance; working with other agencies; monitoring, review and evaluating. This latter aspect of the training will, moreover, lay emphasis on 'grounding work in evidence-based practice' (DfEE 2000b: 14). Foundation training will be structured around five areas. Significantly, these 'core elements' also focus on *seeking transformations in other services* as well as in young people. The five areas are somewhat blandly identified as: engaging with young people; working to secure change with young people, their parents and/or carers and practitioners in the mainstream learning environment; securing an optimal response from all agencies in the community in supporting young people through change; demonstrating success, keeping in touch, record keeping, measurement and evaluation; improving service delivery through reflective practice in context (DfEE 2000b: 15).

Extension training programmes will also 'build on' the initial training provided (DfEE 2000b: 16), but the aim is to merge the foundation and extension programmes into entry-level qualification. More fundamental than mere qualifications, however, will be the project of forging a new professional identity. Linked with this process, therefore, will be the creation of a 'national centre', or 'professional college', to enable personal advisers to begin to 'cohere as a profession' (DfEE 2000b: 18). At present it remains unclear whether this institution will be 'actual' or 'virtual', but the 'scope of the centre or college could include other related professionals, advisers and mentors, such as New Deal advisers and learning support assistants within schools' (DfEE 2000b: 18). The institution is likely, however, to 'promote key principles which underlie the personal adviser role and cover areas such as multidisciplinary practice and management, community involvement and links with neighbourhood renewal, equal opportunities and the promotion of evidence-based practice' (DfEE 2000b: 18).

The role being mapped out for the personal adviser, therefore, encompasses a range of tasks and duties, which both overlap and potentially impinge on roles at present being fulfilled by staff in other agencies. This may be particularly significant in terms of the impact on local authority social work with children and families, because, as observed earlier, social work is *already* being bypassed by a number of New Labour initiatives targeted at children and families.

Inspiration, exhortation and compulsion

The cultural transformations being promoted within and across the new agencies and services working with children and families are, however, just as fundamental as the organisational transitions (see also Hall 1993, 1998).

As observed, although remaining a public agency, the Connexions Service and personal advisers will, like the Youth Justice Board and the Youth Offending Teams, be beyond more traditional departmental bureaucratic structures (Ainsley *et al.* 2002). These agencies, with their commitment to 'what works' and 'evidenced-based practice' are also, in sense, beyond ideology (see also Macdonald and Roberts 1995; Atherton 1999; Hodgkinson 2000; Webb 2001). The Connexions Service and the personal advisers will, for example, have a new identity, a new *esprit de corps*, and the new 'brand' or ambience, heavily influenced by discourses and practices in the United States, is clearly important (McGregor 1999). Particular attention is given over to the inspirational qualities of the agency employee, with mentoring playing a significant role in structuring and organising internal corporate *mores* and cultures and influencing how the agency relates to the users of services.

Helen Colley (2001) has noted that there are no empirical studies of mentoring in the United Kingdom which provide evidence of the 'mind set' of mentors in relation to the young people with whom they are involved. There 'is an assumption that mentoring will not only create "filter-down" benefits such as self confidence and higher aspirations for socially excluded young people, but also that it will create tolerance and a sense of social solidarity' (Colley 2001: 3). Her own fascinating investigations reveal, however, that the views of some mentors are disparaging of the class background of the many young people in need of help. Despite research such as this, the government remains keen on the role mentors can play. This, moreover, has been explicitly connected with how they can provide 'the right role models for boys with absent fathers' and help restore affective bonds inside communities (Ministerial Group on the Family 1998: 15–16; see also Etzioni 1995; Campbell 1995b). In 1998, for example, the then Home Secretary, Jack Straw, spoke nostalgically of the days when the 'lad who previously could not aspire to a university education would aspire to a craft, and gained much from the *tutelage of older men*' (in Vaughan 2000: 349, emphasis added; see also Bruegel 2000).

Certainly a new emphasis is being placed on the 'personal charisma' of this phalanx of mentors and 'enforcement counsellors' who staff the new agencies of the Third Way (Jordan 2000: 29; 14; see also Butler and Drakeford 2001). As suggested, in previous chapters, this is partly rooted in US approaches to social and welfare policy and it is again apparent in the literature centred on the Connexions Service and Youth Offending Teams (see also 'Charismatic staff in Southwark', *Youth Justice Board News*, September 2002: 5). Knowledge, experience and understanding will not suffice because the 'emergent new professional' must also be streetwise, tough and – most important – inspirational and skilled in the arts of exhortation (see also Vaughan 2000: 354). Much of this relates to a new political, social and cultural emphasis on voluntarism and a post-Marxist contempt for anything resembling a materialist interpretation of social dynamics (see Garrett 2003b). However, this promotion of 'people changers' (in Jordan 2000: 15), such as personal advisers and their satellite mentors, can also be associated with the more embedded 'can do' ethos of the American market economy and the more recent popularity of particular variants of managerialism (Pollitt 1993; Clarke and Newman 1997). None of this is to argue, of course, that personal charisma and inspirational qualities have not previously been prized in social work with children and families, but it is to maintain that a fresh and different type of emphasis is being placed on these qualities in the new welfare domains of the Third Way (Neocleous 1999; Jordan 2000; Powell 1999, 2000).[2]

Another dimension of the role of the personal adviser and mentors can be associated with New Labour's more general orientation to social and welfare policy where *advice* frequently blurs into *compulsion*. This approach to welfare is most apparent in relation to employment and benefit entitlement, but it can also be identified in other areas of the welfare state (Butler and Drakeford 2001). In 2001, for example, Jobseekers' Allowance began to be withdrawn from some claimants, in one particular 'pathfinder area', if they refused to heed the *advice* that their literacy and numeracy skills needed improving because this was, it was claimed, undermining their employability. So, for example; 'ES [Employment Services] will provide *advice*, encouragement and courses to support the client, but in return the *client will be expected to* participate in an independent basic skills assessment and any provision that assessment recommends or risk losing benefit' (DfEE 2001d, emphases added). The point here is that this authoritarian dynamic could also begin to inform micro-engagements between personal advisers, mentors and young people and other professionals, such as social workers (see also Mead 1997).

Having briefly outlined the new agency and the role of personal advisers and gone on to look at some of the possible implications for social work with children and families, we will now briefly examine some of the discourses which are embedded in the Connexions literature. These are frequently enmeshed, but can, for heuristic purposes, be separated out and identified as centred on: youth transitions; social exclusion and disaffection; risk; and youth surveillance. Other discourses pivoting on, for example, the 'cycle of disadvantage' can also be located, but it is to these four thematic preoccupations that we shall now turn. These discourses are important for the Connexions Service, but they are also likely to influence *all* multidisciplinary endeavours involving the agency and personal advisers.

Making connections

One of the chief preoccupations of Connexions is youth employment, or what is more commonly referred to as 'the world of work'. This aim of ensuring that employment, education and Welfare services *produce* young citizens who will *fit* is, of course, reflected in the New Deal (DfEE 2001b, c). As we saw in earlier chapters, this concern is also apparent in the LAC system's scrutiny of the so-called 'social presentation' of young care leavers – and managers' responses to it – and in muddled initiatives such as the Quality Protects – Teenagers to Work Day held in April 2000 (see also Beder 2000).

Such an approach to 'the world of work' – that is, to the induction of young people into employment relations primarily structured and organised around the needs of capital – is implicitly informed by social functionalism (Prideaux 2001; see also Klein 2000; Taylor 1999: ch. 2). Furthermore, this dominant orientation is now given additional impetus – and at times a nationalist edge – in the context of concern about the impact of 'globalisation' and the threat from 'competitor' economies also engaged in the relentless struggle for capital accumulation (DfEE 2000a: 16; see also Bauman 1998; Sivanandan 1998/9; Yeates 1999; Jameson 2000; Fitzpatrick 2001; Harris 2001). It is asserted, for example, that it 'is vital, if we are to *succeed as a nation*, and if our young people are to succeed as individuals in the knowledge economy of the twenty-first century . . . [then] we must provide all teenagers with the opportunity and support they need to make the transition to adulthood' (DfEE 2000a: 8, emphasis added). Meanwhile the Prime Minister has spoken of the aim of achieving 'a better life for young people . . . saving them from the prospect of dead-end jobs . . . The Connexions strategy will, therefore, provide the best possible support in the transition from adolescence to adulthood' (Blair in DfEE 2000c, emphases added).

For Fergusson *et al.* (2000) both these statements can also be located within a 'transitions discourse'. During the past twenty years, as can be observed with the LAC materials for older children, this has been *the* dominant discourse for interpreting the experiences of the vast majority of thirteen to nineteen-year-olds (see also Furlong and Cartmel 1997). Within this frame of reference, it is argued, this is a period which 'constitutes a linear transition from school to employment or further education/ higher education. The objectifiable rationality of the process is secured principally through the judgements, assessments and interventions of teachers and careers staff operating within a classic bureau-professional mode' (Fergusson *et al.* 2000: 31). In this way, therefore, the Connexions Service can be seen to represent a reinvigoration of this approach, with personal advisers available to assist young people to make 'realistic choices' and 'right decisions' (DfEE 2000c: 8).

The Connexions Service can, however, also be interpreted as being motivated by another discourse which is 'largely a product of the massive contraction of youth labour markets' (Fergusson *et al.* 2000: 33; see also Bruegel 2000). This is the discourse of social exclusion and disaffection (see also Byrne 1999). Thus the Connexions Service strategy is partly pre-occupied with the need to 'combat civic disengagement' (DfEE 2000a: 15) and a desire to promote organic links between 'teenagers' and 'community', to help the former to become 'active citizens – adults to be proud of' (Blunkett in DfEE 2000a: 8; see also Home Office 2001). In this context, ideas that New Labour is 'developing' include 'summer activities' for all sixteen-year-olds before they take up post-sixteen education, traineeships or work with training (DfEE 2000a: 12). Young people can 'benefit from the experience of positive activity, which could include a summer camp aimed at developing team work, interpersonal skills and leadership' (DfEE 2000a: 12). Perhaps such ideas emphasise what has been termed the 'curriculisation' of the lives of young people (Ennew 1994: 127) and, once again, indicate US influences. However, they can also be related to the third key discourse embedded in Connexions, which centred on risk.

The summer after compulsory education is, we are advised, a 'key transition point when many young people are *vulnerable and at risk* of dropping out of learning, and so excluding themselves from future opportunities' (DfEE 2000a: 12, emphasis added). Risk is, of course, a key sociological trope in Western intellectual debates in the early twenty-first century (Beck 1998; Rustin 1994; Dingwell 1999; O'Brien et al. 1999; Rose 2000; Taylor-Gooby 2001). What is striking, however, is the sheer prominence given to risk in the Connexions literature (see also Furlong and Cartmel 1997). In short, young people are consistently presented as being precariously positioned on life's 'pathway' (DfEE 2000a: 17; see also Prideaux 2001: 89–90). They are, for example, 'at risk of disaffection' (DfEE 2000a: 17): 'at risk of not participating in education and training' (DfEE 2000a: 38); 'at risk of underachieving' (DfEE 2000a: 44) and so on (see also Social Exclusion Unit 1999: part 1). Elsewhere, we are advised that Connexions is now reaching young people who previously 'slipped through the net' because now the 'net is so small that no young person falls through' (DfEE 2001d: 10). All this suggests the vulnerability of youth, with the valiant personal adviser as Salinger's Holden Caulfield having to 'come out from somewhere and catch them'.[3] None the less, the idea of the 'net so small that no young person falls through' can be interpreted in a less benign way, particularly in the context of the sophisticated tracking devices which are evolving as part of the Connexions package. This aspect of the new agency, its strategy and practices, can be understood within a discourse of youth surveillance.

Connexions, surveillance and strategies of virtual control

The Connexions Service will maintain a database and we are advised that its aim is 'to ensure that the agency is aware of all young people and their education, training or employment status . . . It will allow monitoring of the help provided to those not in learning *or at risk of becoming dis-connected from their current learning or work*' (DfEE 2000a: 57, emphasis added). Elsewhere this database is referred to as a 'register' of the entire population of thirteen to nineteen-year-olds in every area which will furnish details of 'learning progress, current status *and other information needed by personal advisers*' (DfEE 2000c: 9). Partially alert to the impact on civil liberties of this type of mass logging, monitoring and surveillance activity, it is unconvincingly stated that 'advisers *or specialists* dealing with an individual will be able to access *relevant* information about that young person, with clear protocols covering data exchange and access' (DfEE 2000c: 9, emphases added).

Some are fairly relaxed about this development and perceive tracking activity as largely to the advantage of the 'vulnerable' young who may be at 'risk' (see, for example, Canny *et al.* 2001; Green *et al.* 2001). However, concern has already been expressed, particularly in Chapter 2, about the extent of information flows and the collation and exchange of information on young people who are 'looked after' (see also Rose 2000). In addition, there are more general fears about how technological innovations, such as computer databases, enhance the surveillance capacity of the state and multinational corporations (Dandeker 1990; Poster 1990; Wilson 1999; Haggerty and Ericson 2000). Bloomfield (2001: 175), for example, has suggested that certain movements 'in time and space present a potential problem of social order/disorder' and 'new regimes of virtual control . . . are directed at solving the (supposed) deficit in order or threats posed to it'. The suggestion here is that these remarks have particular resonance in relation to the CS database and the Connexions card – or so-called 'smart card' – to be discussed later. In order to try to comprehend why this is so, it is necessary, therefore, to briefly refer to the social and professional context in which these 'new regimes of virtual control' are increasingly being deployed.

Historically, of course, *some* young people have always been perceived as a threat to the social order (Hendrick 1994). However, as we saw in Chapter 2, from the early 1980s onwards these fears became more emphatic and focused on, for example, the alleged loss of 'childhood innocence', the 'end of the family', 'fatherless families', a growing 'underclass' or 'new rabble' and the alleged incompetence of social services staff in 'containing' and 'managing' 'looked after' young people (see Murray 1990, 1994; Straw and Anderson 1996; Scraton 1997; Morgan 1999). Partly as a result, a range of measures have been put in place to 'deal with' young offenders and *potential* young offenders (Home Office 2000; Youth Justice Board 2001a, b; James and James 2001; see also 'Nurseries seek power to expel violent toddlers', *The Independent*, 12 April 2001). Furthermore, electronic technologies are beginning to play a much more prominent role in regulating this section of the population (see also 'Tags and VoiceTrack –

the positive alternative to custody', *Youth Justice Board News* 4, June 2000: 2; 'Virtual conferences are a hit', *Youth Justice Board News* 8, June 2001: 11; 'Mobiles join fight against truancy', *The Guardian*, 1 June 2001). None of this is to imply that electronic technologies cannot play a socially beneficial role (see Bloomfield 2001). The aim is simply to highlight potentially problematic aspects of the CS desire to constantly 'keep in touch' with thirteen to nineteen-year-olds. Indeed, the database, or 'register', can be perceived as liable to be abused in the context of multidisciplinary working, particularly as it relates to 'troublesome' young people. However, it is the Connexions card, which should, perhaps, give social workers and others in social care the greatest cause for concern.

From August 2001 children between the ages of thirteen and nineteen began to be issued with the Connexions card. Essentially it is an identity card for 2.4 million young people, but its attraction, for the young, is that possession of it can provide discounts on cinema tickets, travel and other goods and services. This is because young people 'will be able to earn reward points for *positive* activities related to learning (for example regular attendance) which can be redeemed in a wide range of retail outlets' (DfEE 2000a: 24, emphasis added). This also emphasises, of course, the public/private mix underpinning Connexions and other New Labour innovations. The newsletter 'for everyone working in' the Connexions Service coyly confides, for example, that 'apart from attracting new customers, organisations are hoping to use the card to raise their profile in the local community and indeed promote the company as a careers option' (*Making Connexions* 1, March 2001: 4). More fundamentally, of course, the card enables commercial sponsors to *target* young consumers.

Integral to the card is a 'smart' facility which can be used to monitor and check attendance on courses, pay for education-related expenses and, as we have seen, earn 'points' following the completion of training, education or voluntary work. One 'demonstration project', for example, has already used the 'attendance monitoring system to test benefits in relation to tracking and validating Education Maintenance Allowance eligibility and rewards and loyalty functions' (DfEE 2000a: 14). Unsurprisingly, the Connexions Service has had to listen to young people's concerns about the card (*Making Connexions* 1, March 2001: 2). However, these worries are not satisfactorily addressed and it is merely proclaimed that the introduction of the card will be the 'largest rollout of a smart card in an open environment anywhere in the world' (*Making Connexions* 1, March 2001: 4). Moreover, concern about the impact on civil liberties is treated in a derisory way. A couple of pages after quickly alluding to the concerns of young people, it is simply reported in bold lettering: 'The Connexions Card scheme will be an excellent opportunity for students to really experience the rewards that learning and education can offer, as well as being able to watch rugby more easily and affordably' (*Making Connexions* 1, March 2001: 4).

This trite response to serious concern can, perhaps, also be associated with a more embedded failure to engage with children, families and communities about Connexions. Despite references to 'listening' to young people, it is clear that the entire Connexions strategy is very much a 'top-down' strategy (see also, however, DfEE 2001e). Thus the Connexions Service will 'reach down into communities' and a guide is being produced 'so that local communities and voluntary organisations *know what is happening*' (DfEE 2000c: 4, emphasis added). Despite such an approach, liberal professions, such as social work, need to question the discourse of youth surveillance which underpins the 'register' and the Connexions card. Many young users of social services, subject already to what Lindsay (1998) terms 'careism', are likely to be rendered especially visible by the new means of electronic surveillance which the Connexions Service is to deploy. Moreover, the crude behavioural approach represented by the 'rewards' dimension needs to be responded to with the utmost caution (see also Peck 1998: 135; 'Blair's CD ploy to reclaim the streets', *The Guardian*, 25 April 2001).

As we can see, therefore, a range of factors indicates that the Connexions enterprise needs to be looked at in some detail. It is not simply that social workers should be fearful for their jobs, or alert to defend 'their' professional territory. However, the final part of the chapter will briefly look at how the growth in the number of personal advisers and mentors may, indeed, impact on social work recruitment.

'Social work – it's all about people': connexions and the social work recruitment crisis[4]

In England, since 1995, there has been a 15 per cent increase in social services staff working with children (Department of Health 2001g: 9). However, figures released by the Department of Health reveal that social services posts, in total, decreased by 2 per cent between September 1999 and September 2000 and by 7 per cent since September 1995. The sharpest fall was in residential care posts: 18 per cent lower than 1995 (Department of Health 2001g: 1). Across the Social Services Department sector, as a whole, there are also fears, in some quarters, that Health, under the guise of NHS Care Trusts, is beginning to 'take over' parts of Social Services Departments (Burrows 2001). Evidence is also beginning to emerge of social services staff being 'lured away' by the better salaries, terms and conditions in parts of the Health Service (Winchester 2001b; see also 'Staff see an end to Social Services Departments', *Community Care*, 31 May–6 June 2001: 3).

135

These developments provide, therefore, part of the context for the evolution of the Connexions Service. Indeed, it is clear that personal advisers and mentors, many of uncertain purpose and function, will continue to swim into those fluid spaces, which now characterises the amorphous world of social work and social care. Specifically in relation to the impact of the Connexions Service on Social Services Departments, a recruitment drive to widen the pool of personal advisers is, therefore, likely to further deplete the numbers of social workers and potential social workers currently available.[5] Certainly the salaries available for personal advisers are likely to induce some social workers to consider a move to the Connexions Service, given that after 'a mere 150 hours (about a month) of training, full-time personal advisers will earn anything between £15,000 and £35,000, sometimes with a car thrown in' (Winchester 2001a: 19).

More broadly, concerns existed, of course, about the decline in inquiries about social work training and applications to social work courses even in the early 1990s. However, pleas from ADSS for a 'coherent, national approach to recruitment' were rejected by successive Conservative administrations (see 'Social work recruits plea', *The Guardian*, 29 September 1990). In 2000 a number of local authorities began to recruit staff from Australia, Canada and South Africa. This resulted in, largely ignored, protests from the South African government ('South African Minister attacks poaching of staff', *Community Care*, 31 May–6 June 2001: 8; 'UK recruitment agency sets up shop in Pretoria', *Community Care*, 14–20 June 2001: 5). Indeed, as Bill Jordan (2001: 529) suggested, the 'drive to import child protection workers (along with teachers and nurses)' could result in 'ideal recruits for New Labour's public service regime' because they are 'mostly young, single and willing to tolerate spartan accommodation' (see also Eden *et al.* 2002). None the less, because of the sheer scale of the recruitment crisis, with the Local Government Association (LGA) suggesting that 63 per cent of local authorities were struggling to recruit social workers, New Labour launched a national recruitment drive.

However, unlike similar recruitment drives for nurses and teachers which offered additional money to attract people, the social work initiative has largely focused on trying to improve the 'image' of the profession (see also Jerrom 2001).[6] This was, therefore, the emphasis of a national newspaper and radio advertising campaign, which began in October 2001. The message of the campaign was somewhat blurred, though, when the Health Secretary used the official launch of the recruitment drive to name and lambast England's ten 'worst performing' Social Services Departments (see the editorial 'Milburn out of touch', *Community Care*, 25–31 October 2001: 5). More fundamentally, the literature and dominant representations produced in association with the recruitment drive can be interpreted as portraying the world in a shallow and depoliticised way. This, moreover, is particularly the case in relation to a series of comic strip vignettes which appeared in the national press.

As can be seen from the frontispiece of this book, each vignette, constructed like a storyboard outline for a film, was accompanied by the bland phrase 'People can be fascinating, mystifying, rewarding. They're never boring'. This was then used as the foundation of a short narrative in which the reader (or potential social work recruit) was presented as being able to intervene to promote a better life for the vignette's focal individual (for example, an autistic child, an elderly Polish man who has survived a concentration camp). These encounters, involving social workers, appear almost magical and this is reinforced by the golden glow surrounding the pictorial imagery. No sense is conveyed of the complexity of people's hardships, or that the users of social services exist in structural locations where issues such as poverty impinge. Neither is there any indication that the social worker is part of a wider welfare bureaucracy. Indeed, the adverts, with their shallow and facile resolution of profound and intractable human problems, merely recall the more mawkish of Hollywood films.

Conclusion

It has been argued that it is 'alarming just how unaware many health and social care staff, youth workers and education welfare staff are of Connexions, the enormous steamroller bearing down on them' (Winchester 2001a: 18). Indeed, perhaps most comment so far has concentrated on the impact of the Connexions Service on, for example, youth work (Ansell 2001; see also, however, Higham 2001). The argument in this chapter is that the Connexions Service needs to be interrogated because of its possible impact on young users of social services and on social work with children and families more generally.

9

CONCLUSION

Clearly, social work is always, in a sense, being *remade* and it is not possible to have nervous recourse to an authentic or timeless form of practice. Social work is always changing and evolving into something else, always *in process*. However, what, at present, can we say about the current shape and trajectory of social work with children and families?

New structures and new professions

A key change clearly relates to the promotion of multidisciplinary working and 'joined up' approaches to social work with children and families (see Local Government Association, NHS Confederation, ADSS 2002). More emphatically, the Department of Health has maintained that 'sustained investment in social services' will require the 'breaking down of the "Berlin wall" that divides health and social services' (Department of Health 2002e; see also Leason 2002).

In October 2002 the Health Secretary, Alan Milburn (2002), made it clear that he wanted more 'radical' changes when he asserted that 'old-style public service monoliths cannot meet modern challenges. They need to be broken up.' He also envisaged the creation of Children's Trusts and called on the GSCC and associated bodies to work towards the creation of 'new types of social care professionals'. He specifically referred to 'family care workers' who would combine the 'skills of health visitors and social workers to provide support in [rather ambiguously] times of trouble' (see also the editorial 'The end of social workers', *Community Care*, 31 October–6 November 2002: 5).

These plans for 'new professionals' in the area of social care have also been promoted by others seeking to influence the New Labour agenda (see, particularly, Kendall and Harker 2002). Elsewhere, we have seen, as discussed earlier, the arrival of the 'emergent new professional', the personal adviser, who is at the fulcrum of Connexions. In addition, new agencies such as Youth Offending Teams and Sure Start projects are becoming more central in policy and in practice.

Direction from the centre

Irrespective of the organisational forms, which will emerge in the next few years, it is apparent that New Labour, like its Conservative predecessors, will continue to extend control over both the *processes* and the *outputs* of what we currently regard as social work with children and families. In other areas of the public sector similar moves have, of course, also taken place (see Newman 2001: ch. 5). In terms of changes introduced having an impact on processes, social work with children and families is becoming a heavily prescribed activity which is increasingly dominated by centrally devised schedules, such as the LAC materials and the more recently introduced *Framework for the Assessment of Children in Need and their Families*. These assessment 'tools' are similar in that they provide evidence of a new, or reinvigorated, form of Taylorism (in this context see also Fox 1993: 47–9). Harrison (2002) has detected similar developments in health-care organisations. However, it is also important to view changes in social work and social care labour processes alongside more pervasive transformations taking place across the 'world of work'. In this context, Bain *et al.* (2002: 172) in their research on the expanding 'call centre' sector have referred to management's 'desire to set targets to measure not only the "hard", quantitative aspects of an employees' tasks, but also to exert more control and direction over the performance of those "soft", qualitative areas of employee–customer interaction'. The argument is not, of course, that changes to labour processes in social work and other areas of social care are simply mirroring those taking place in other sectors. However, our awareness of changes in ostensibly entirely different work domains can aid our understanding of transitions taking place in social work and associated areas.

More fundamentally, the argument is that there remains a need to be wary about schedules, instruments, frameworks and other centrally devised documentation which seek to entirely structure and organise the manner of engagement with children and families. Social workers are not automata, but there may be an inclination to 'keep to the official definition of the situation and not to move beyond the constraints imposed by protocol and procedures' (Spratt and Houston 1999: 320). In some respects, a challenge to the use of particular sets of forms – or even *specific* questions posed on forms – can be perceived as a more fundamental questioning of the 'way things are around here'. For individual workers this can result in pressure from more malleable colleagues and from managers in the workplace (see Gubruim *et al.* 1989: 212). None the less, critical analysis and creative work need to take place in order to resist proceduralisation and the imposition of bureaucratic constraints which frequently seek to produce manageable, docile social technicians and compliant users of services. Perhaps there also needs to be renewed counter-emphasis on the importance of non-directed 'talk' and 'conversation' in social work encounters (see Parton and O'Byrne 2000).[1] Significantly, this would also seem to gel with parents' views of what makes a 'good social worker'. Research has indicated that their emphasis is on approachability, honesty, having time to listen, understanding, reliability and helpfulness (Aldgate and Statham 2001: 79–82). Conspicuously absent from this list was a social worker's proficiency in completing the Family Pack of Questionnaires and Scales (Department of Health, Cox and Bentovim 2000).

It's in the stars: targets and social work in a 'performative society'

The fixation on outputs, evidenced by the plethora of 'targets', league tables and performance indicators which it is maintained will improve 'outcomes' for children, has also been a significant and highly ambiguous development, which has taken place during the period discussed in this book. In spring 2002, for example, a 'new star rating system' was introduced which 'brings together all the existing performance data' across services for children and adults (Platt 2002: 36). A number of local authorities which received 'zero ratings' have undergone a regime change and are being 'assisted' by multinational corporate management consultants. Thus, at the time of writing, Price Waterhouse Coopers is developing a children's strategy for north-east Lincolnshire. In Birmingham, Deloitte & Touche are 'assisting' in improving the review system for children who are 'looked after' and children on the child protection register. Meanwhile the consultancy firm of Klynveld Peat Marwick Goerdeler (KPMG) is doing similar work in Walsall and Coventry (Hunter 2002). In contrast, those local authorities deemed to be doing well, 'three-star councils', will have 'available to them a series of "freedoms"' and will be able to access a Performance Fund (SSI 2002).

Social services are publicly owned and there should be systems in place which render their work visible to those who pay for and use services (see also Coote 2002). However, leaving aside the imposition of the management consultants, there are fundamental problems with the entire 'star rating' scheme. It seeks, for example, with its allocation of 'stars', to transplant the vocabulary and orientation more readily associated with the market, particularly those market niches concerned with the consumption of leisure products, into the field of social care. Furthermore, the Comprehensive Performance Assessment (CPA) which the star ratings feed into will result in local authorities being presented with 'annual report cards'. This, it might be argued, seeks to infantilise democratically elected local councils. The fact that the CPA will also situate councils in one of four streams – top performing, striving, coasting or failing – also serves to emphasise the sheer banality of this managerialist approach.

In a more abstract sense, Ball (2001), who draws on the work of Foucault, Lyotard and Deleuze, has emphasised the significance of 'performativity' in education, but his contribution is also applicable to and aids our analysis of the remaking of social work with children and families. Central to Ball's argument is the emergence of what he dubs personal and institutional *fabrications*. These are 'versions of an organisation (or person) which do not exist – they are not "outside the truth" but neither do they render simply true or direct accounts – they are produced purposely in order "to be accountable"'(Ball 2001: 218). These fabrications are then apt to become embedded in and reproduced by systems of recording and reporting on practice. New Labour's naive managerialist faith in star ratings and other means of trying to render complex organisations 'accountable' and 'transparent' fails to incorporate any sense of the dynamics of performativity and the representational fabrications associated with it (see also Rose 1993, 1996). Returning specifically to social work with children and families, the Social Services Department primarily responsible for the welfare of Victoria Climbié received a 'glowing joint review' just months before the child's death (see the editorial 'Who inspects the reviews?' *Community Care*, 11–17 July 2002: 5). The soundness of this review was, moreover, reinforced in the fourth annual report on joint reviews (Rickford 2002b). Indeed, perhaps, these events provide a tragic illustration of the aptness of Ball's analysis.

Looking forwards, looking backwards: complex 'modernisation'

It would, however, be wrong to view the many changes taking place as conclusive evidence of the evolution of a new, entirely transformed social work. Clearly, social work, in general, is now regulated by a panoply of new quangos and there are also hints, as observed earlier, of a wholesale restructuring with the imminent introduction of Children's Trusts and – possibly – a Child Protection Agency (Downey 2002). The vocabulary of social work and some of its focal conceptualisations is also changing, with, as we have seen, the introduction of thematic notions of 'social exclusion' and 'inclusive practice'. However, elsewhere – even within the discourse of New Labour's 'modernisation' agenda – we can see a reaffirmation of the 'appropriateness' of more embedded approaches to social work with children and families. This can be seen, as indicated earlier, in terms of how the government has attempted to relocate child adoption at the centre of practice.

It remains necessary to be cautious about the political enthusiasm for 'quick fixes' (such as more child adoptions) for complex issues relating to socially and economically marginalised children and families. However, promoting the adoption of 'looked after' children also illuminates how, in the remaking of social work with children and families, historically rooted concerns and preoccupations are being recast to fit the managerialist vision and orientation. This is also apparent with other New Labour initiatives, such as those in relation to 'cutting teenage pregnancies'. Here 'ambitious targets' seek to 'halve the rate of conception in under-18s by 2010, with an interim reduction of 15 per cent by 2004'. In some localities, 'teenage mothers' are also to be 'allocated a dedicated adviser' (in Hayes 2002: 10). This approach highlights New Labour's managerialist fondness for 'measurement'. It also reveals, as argued in Chapter 8, the centrality of a new cadre of mentors and advisers. However, if these fresh elements are stripped away, perhaps at the core of the initiative is an historically rooted and class-based concern about the alleged 'fecklessness' and fecundity of the poor and 'dangerous' classes (see Bosanquet 1895; Haylett 2001a, b). Again focusing on continuities with the past, whilst recognising that the gradual evolution of more sophisticated approaches to monitoring ethnicity are beginning to evolve, it has also been argued, in Chapter 7, that social work largely continues to view the world as 'black' or 'white' and still fails to take adequate account of the diversity *within* these essentialist categories.

New Labour's 'modernisation' of social work and social care builds, in some respects, on the 'reforms' which began to be introduced in the Major period. However, the Labour administration's remaking of social work is complex and far from unidirectional. In some quarters, for example, there are even hints of wariness about the use of 'checklists'. In 2002 the Chief Inspector of Social Services also championed, albeit in fairly ambiguous terms, a 'culture of care, which puts an end to checklists that replace thinking and judgement' (SSI 2001: 7). Elsewhere, within the DoH literature there has been a rediscovery of the 'processes of psycho-social casework' (Aldgate and Statham 2001: 136). In a theoretical sense, Susan White (1998b: 264) has also challenged the view that the 'traditional dominance of psychological and developmental forms of thought in child welfare is being eroded'. Consequently, for her, 'rumours of the waning of the "psy" complex have been greatly exaggerated' (White 1998b: 266; see also Rose 1985). Indeed, the LAC materials are grounded in developmental theory and this relates to a further observation:

> The assessment checklists, which are an increasing feature of child welfare practice, have incorporated a bastardized scientific knowledge, translated by policy makers, child welfare professionals and

by the juridical field into *technical instruments which promise the truth.*

(White 1998b: 279, emphasis added)

The introduction of a new social work degree is, of course, also likely to have an impact on how social work with children and families evolves.

New Labour, the new degree and 'practical' social work

In May 2002 the Department of Health announced the details of the curriculum for this new social work degree. The aim of the new award was to 'prepare students for the reality of becoming a social worker' (Department of Health 2002b). The title of the press release accompanying the announcement was, however, revealing: 'New social work degree will focus on practical training'. The Health Minister, Jacqui Smith, elaborated:

> Social work is a very practical job. It is about protecting people and changing their lives, not about being able to give fluent and theoretical explanations about why they got into difficulties in the first place. [See also Philpot 2002.]

There is, however, a need to try and promote a critical agenda in social work with children and families – to go beyond the 'practical' and to constantly ask not only *how*, but also *why*. Indeed, this view is reaffirmed in the Department of Health's own literature on social work education. Barnes (2002: 13) in her interviews with focus groups on the future of social work training found that there 'was a need for courses to develop curricula which will ensure that students acquire knowledge about the origins and development of those social problems which are routinely likely to encounter and strategies to deal with them'. However, there were 'shortfalls' in relation to students' 'knowledge of the origins of social problems'. Social work students, according to Barnes (2002: 12) tend to simply interpret 'knowledge' as 'gathering information about people'.

In terms of trying to understand 'social problems', social work should, perhaps, be a little more willing to integrate class and facets of Marxist approaches into its analytical frameworks (see Jones 1997; also Harvey 2002; Houston 2002). Capitalism 'without classes is inconceivable' (Furlong and Cartmel 1997: 112) and class remains central to the life chances (the 'outcomes') of those who use social services. The warranted concern about, for example, the health status of children and young people 'looked after' (Butler and Payne 1997) inescapably relates not only to specific factors associated with the experience of being 'looked after' but also connects, in quite profound ways, with their social class location (Bebbington and Miles 1989; see also Jordan 2000: 101). In relation to the LAC materials, some of the young people interviewed about the implementation of the system in Scotland also 'identified what they felt was a broader agenda, a class bias, that did not reflect their backgrounds or circumstances' (Francis 2002: 457). All this suggests that social work education, for example, needs to begin to acknowledge the centrality of class. As Beverley Skeggs (1997: 6–7), in her fascinating study of the relationship between gender and class, has asserted:

> the retreat from class has occurred across a range of academic sites. [However] when a retreat is mounted we need to ask whose experiences are being silenced, whose lives are being ignored and whose lives are considered worthy of study. We also need to think about the relationship between responsibility and knowledge: to ignore, or make class invisible is to abdicate responsibility (through privilege) from the effects it produces. [See also Gamble *et al.* 1999 and 'Social class key to children's success', *The Guardian*, 9 August 2002.]

This is not, of course, to 'reduce the social field, a multidimensional space, to the economic field alone, to the relations of economic production' (Bourdieu 1991: 231). More specifically, it is not to deny the validity of other social divisions rooted in, for example, gender, generation, 'race' and ethnicity. It is, however, to suggest that these other social divisions and cleavages cannot – analytically or in terms of lived experience – be understood without encompassing the economic dimension. This point also relates to one of the book's constantly recurring themes: the explicit and implicit acceptance of existing economic relations (and what is sometimes referred to as 'the world of work') in the 'tools' devised for social work practice. The functionalist orientation of these 'tools' – and the associated documentation – frequently seek, in fact, to merely contribute to the shaping of well presented employees who are able to 'fit' into their allocated space in a market economy. Coupled with this is the deepening of social authoritarianism, reflected in the Framework's Core Assessment Record, which inquires, as we have seen, whether the parents' relationship with 'those in authority' is generally 'harmonious'.

Social work and human rights in a 'surveillance society'

Another major theme which has emerged in this book relates to how the remaking of social work with children and families cannot be detached from the gradual criminalisation of child welfare discourses. This was revealed, for example, in Chapter 4, where within joint social work/police child protection teams the social work role appeared to become 'blurred', with, in some instances, the social work dimension being subject to what was termed 'voluntary liquidation'. There are also some indications that the direction of the Youth Justice Board is increasingly being steered by the police. In late 2002, for example, it was announced that 'as part of the YJB's commitment to improving the performance and quality of its service' the new role of Regional Manager was to be created. Of the eight selected, two are former police chief superintendents and one is a seconded prison governor (see 'Regional Managers to take up their posts', *Youth Justice Board News*, December 2002: 5).

Related to this, since the early 1990s we have seen a renewed emphasis on the need to detect the alleged crimogenic proclivities of the children of the unemployed and working poor. This trend, associated with 'multi-disciplinary working' and 'joined-up thinking', can be related to the state, in all its myriad forms, increasingly seeking to enhance its surveillance capacity. A constellation of factors – including technological transformations, genetic determinism, a regressive political belief in the efficacy of incarceration and the events of 11 September 2001 – now provide, in differing degrees, part of the foundation for this development, which is more and more impinging on social work and related fields.[2]

In late 2001, for example, and serving to further emphasise some of the developments discussed in Chapters 2 and 8, it was reported that the Metropolitan Police would be piloting a new scheme in eleven London boroughs. The aim was to expand it nationally. At the heart of the plan, reported *ChildRight*, was the establishment of a database listing the names of children [the Metropolitan Police] *believe* may grow up to become 'criminal' (emphasis added). The report went on:

> Children who behave badly or commit minor misdemeanours will be placed on the register and monitored and supervised throughout their childhood. Children as young as three will be included on the database if the police, social services or schools believe they are at risk of committing a crime. In particular, children involved in cheekiness, minor vandalism and causing nuisances will be targeted and they will then be monitored at school and on the streets, despite not having committed a crime.
>
> ('Database for badly behaved children', *ChildRight* 182, December 2001: 2; see also 'Alarm at Met database on likely criminals', *The Guardian*, 22 January 2002)

Some of these ideas have subsequently been incorporated into YJB plans for 'youth inclusion and support panels'. Initially, ten of these multi-disciplinary panels are to be introduced into 'high-level crime areas' in order to identify eight to thirteen-year-olds who are displaying 'problem behaviours'. The Children and Young People's unit is also intent on introducing an information-sharing system for 'at risk' children, known as

Identification, Referral and Tracking (IRT) (Jerrom 2002a). This is expected to be operational by April 2003, yet there has been no piloting and no formal consultation with children and young people. With crime increasingly being used 'as the hook for children's policies' (Rickford 2002c), the criminalisation of child welfare discourses has also been illuminated in *Scotland's Action Programme to Reduce Youth Crime*. This proposed a 'closer integration between the youth justice system and an authority's service for vulnerable children' and would include the 'development and co-ordination of agencies' databases to identify, at an early stage, children and young people who are at risk of offending' (Scottish Executive 2002: 6). Risk factors were reported to embrace 'displays of aggressive antisocial behaviour and hyperactivity, harsh or neglectful parenting, separation from parents and siblings who are offenders themselves' (Smith 2002).

The argument is not that social work with children and families is becoming *entirely* harnessed to more embracing anti-crime preoccupations within a 'surveillance society' (Lyon 2001a). Within criminology and sociology there are also complex debates as to whether surveillance is centralised, in the Orwellian sense, or whether the growth of surveillance systems is dispersed, decentralised and 'rhizomic', more 'like a creeping plant than a centrally controlled trunk with spreading branches' (Lyon 2001a: 4). The suggestion is simply that these developments, irrespective of the exact character of the form of surveillance, are increasingly beginning to influence and shape aspects of social work and to determine its trajectory.[3] As Cohen (1985: 183) has astutely noted, ever 'since the case history came into being, the people-processing professions have received a collective licence for gathering information'. In the early twenty-first century, however, it seems necessary for social work – unsentimentally, a 'people-processing profession' – to seriously reflect on the civil liberties aspect of information gathering and associated practices which frequently seek to restrict the freedoms of children and young people (see also Walsh 2002). Indeed, there are already indications that the evolving Integrated Children's System (ICS) is likely to renew the concern of many about the use of computer-based systems and compilation of electronic databases within Social Services Departments (see, in this context, Rose 2002: 316). This understanding also relates, of course, to human rights and to the Human Rights Act 1998. Some – with good reason – are sceptical of universalist discourses underpinning such legislation (Webb 2002). Indeed, since the Act was introduced there has, perhaps, been a tendency, in some quarters, to over-emphasise its impact (Williams 2001).[4] However, this book suggests that the pragmatic and political invocation of human rights now needs to become more central in social work with children and families (see also Howard League 2002c).

In summary, *The Remaking of Social Work with Children and Families* has been founded on the principle that social workers and social work educators *have to* be prepared to embrace change. However, whilst being willing to be constructively engaged with, for example, some aspects of the 'modernisation' agenda, there is a need to be critical agents in the process of change. That is to say, there is a need to be reflexive and cautious about some of the rhetoric associated with the remaking of child-care social work. In a more fundamental sense, this is inescapably linked with the need to promote and foster democracy and dialogical exchanges within the sphere of social welfare (see also Mouffe 2000). This perspective is under-pinned by the understanding that it is misguided to view social work as an entirely benign and emancipatory activity. In short, social work with children and families should not be sentimentalised and its function and purpose misunderstood. The book has, therefore, attempted to provide a series of critical snapshots of the changes taking place in this area of social care. Consequently, the aim has been to try and prompt alternative ways of viewing themes and issues, which the mainstream, or 'official', dis-courses regard as settled and no longer open to debate or contestation. In these troubled times, however, it remains a democratic imperative to reflect and to question such certainties.

NOTES

1 Introduction

1 Some of the empirical work featured in Chapter 4 was undertaken in Scotland. However, the book will largely discuss developments in England and Wales, where social work with children and families is governed by the Children Act 1989. Perhaps even more specifically, realising that the Welsh Assembly is increasingly able and willing to forge its own policies, the focus will be mostly on England (see also 'Wales goes its own way with NHS reform', *The Guardian*, 15 November 2002).

2 See also 'Social workers make their Soviet debut', *The Guardian*, 17 August 1991. In spring 2002 it was observed in *Community Care* magazine that 'social workers from the UK are being asked in growing numbers to share their skills and expertise to help build a framework for social care in the region [Eastern Europe]. Big funders such as the World Bank are investing in social care in the region and want UK know-how to get it off the ground' (see Rickford 2002a).

3 Throughout the rest of the book the shorthand 'the Framework' will often refer to the *Framework for the Assessment of Children in Need and their Families*.

4 In the United States there have been a number of valuable historical accounts of aspects of social work. See, for example, Tice (1998) whose contribution can be associated with some of the themes in this book.

5 Pauline Marie Rosenau (1992) has identified 'sceptical' and 'affirmative' postmodernists. Within social work, the Australian social work academics Bob Pease and Jan Fook (1999: 12) have drawn a similar distinction. They find themselves 'siding with those expressions of postmodern thinking that do not totally abandon the values of the Enlightenment project of human emancipation. Only "strong" or "extreme" forms of postmodernist theory reject normative criticism and the usefulness of any forms of commonality underlying diversity. We believe that a "weak" form of postmodernism informed by critical theory can contribute effectively to the construction of emancipatory politics concerned with political action and social justice.' It is, however, Peter Leonard (2000) who has been the most persuasive advocate of postmodernist ideas within the field of social work and, more broadly, social welfare. He also maintains that postmodernism is an 'essential ingredient in a revitalised Marxism'.

6 Today there is renewed interest in Taylorism and white-collar work (see, for example, Bain *et al.* 2002). Taylorism refers to the production techniques devised by Frederick W. Taylor (1856–1915) and these were a central component of 'Fordism' (see Harris 1998). There is, of course, a literature which charts and

149

debates the transition from 'Fordist' to 'post-Fordist' organisation of the means of production and distribution (see, for example, Hall and Jacques 1989). Some within the sphere of social care have identified this transition as it relates to their work as, for example, probation officers (see Sparrow *et al.* 2002). Throughout this book, however, there will be no attempt to map out the contours of 'post-Fordist' social work. More fundamentally, we will share Clarke and Newman's (1997) reluctance to present change in terms of 'from–to dualisms'.

7 John Clarke and Janet Newman (1997: 76) have observed that within the discourse of the 'managerialist state' we have seen an 'epidemic of quality'. They relate the omnipresence of this particular word to changes taking place within the public sector. More specifically, a key aim of managerialism is to reshape the place and power of bureau-professionalism (see also Harris 1998). In trying to achieve this aim the promoters of managerialism seek to co-opt bureau-professionals, such as social workers, by colonising the 'terrain of professional discourse, constructing articulations between professional concerns and language and those of management'. Here, therefore, abstract ideas about *quality* appeal to those committed to the maintenance of standards and the dissemination of good practice. However, *quality* can also be interpreted as a 'central mechanism for disciplining professional autonomy'. In terms of social work with children and families, the perfect illustration of this is provided, of course, by New Labour's glibly (but predictably entitled) Quality Protects (QP) programme for children and young people who are 'looked after' (Department of Health 1998b). This clearly appeals to ideas about good practice, yet at the same time it seeks to control, constrain and steer social workers on account of centrally devised benchmarks, which identify and 'measure' the performance of local authorities. John Hopton (1999: 78) has written convincingly of 'quality' as a 'potentially tyrannical concept'. See also the DoH Web site for a list of publications, which have appeared under the rubric of QP, www.doh.gov.uk/qualityprotects/info/publications/index.htm.

8 In February 2002 Prime Minister Tony Blair stated that those who were critical of his faltering project to 'modernise' public services were 'wreckers'. It is, of course, recognised that New Labour is not a monolithic political entity and the Labour Party is a coalition of disparate political currents. In this book, however, New Labour will refer to the Blair administration and to that dominant segment of the parliamentary party which is currently the driving force in remaking social work and other aspects of social welfare in Britain. Chantal Mouffe (2000: 15) has accurately observed that 'Blairism is only conducive to the maintenance of existing hierarchies. No amount of dialogue or preaching will ever convince the ruling class to give up its power.' She concludes that 'Thatcherism with a human face' is the 'trade mark of New Labour' (Mouffe 2000: 119).

PART I MAJOR DEPARTURES?

2 The 'blueprint' for change

1 Later, in Chapter 6, it will be argued that actual parents, or 'birth parents', are also marginalised within the current New Labour approach to the adoption of 'looked after' children.

2 See also the editorial in *Community Care* (28 March–3 April 2002: 5). A survey of 'children in need' in England, undertaken by the Department of Health in September/October 2001, estimated that 2 per cent of those 'looked after' are asylum-seeking children; www.doh.gov.uk/cin/cin2001results.htm.

3 In Chapter 7 it will be suggested that the essentialist categories 'black' and 'white' are not always helpful conceptualisations when engaging with ideas associated with 'race' and ethnicity.

4 Peter Leonard (1997: 1) succinctly defines 'late capitalism' as 'the capitalism of mass consumption within global markets'. This phrase implicitly acknowledges the dynamic elements within capitalism. Indeed, one of the main characteristics of capitalism is the ability to constantly transform itself. 'Capitalism in the general sense is capable of assuming highly variable forms, which continue to be capitalist through the continuity of a number of central features (wage labour, competition, private property, orientation to capital accumulation, technical progress, the rampant commodification of all social activities)' (Chiapello and Fairclough 2002: 187). From October 2002 the national minimum wage for workers aged eighteen to twenty-one was just £3.60 per hour. No minimum wage protection was available for those aged sixteen to seventeen years.

5 This is also reflected in the 'Teenagers to work' initiative launched on 19 April 2000 which was set up under the auspices of New Labour's Quality Protects initiative. Building on the 'National Take your Daughters to Work Day', this was supposed to give 'looked after' children a 'positive experience of work'. Literature associated with the scheme blandly explained that the 'underlying aim is to give young people the opportunity to achieve in the world of work'. On one level this can, of course, be interpreted as entirely benign and 'helpful'. However, the suggestion is that such 'initiatives' can also be interpreted in a more expansive and critical way. Some of these themes will be returned to in Chapter 8.

3 Examining the 'product champions'

1 Information made available at a DoH-hosted conference on the Integrated Children's System (ICS), held in February 2002, revealed how AARs are not being used as the academic researchers and senior civil servants hope that they would be used. This is also clear from briefing papers produced on the ICS. It is revealed, for example, that AARs are 'used in about 40 per cent of appropriate cases. Moreover, they are only rarely used on a routine basis'. In a 'longitudinal cohort study, after two years of follow-up about 60 per cent of the children had one AAR on file, but only 13 per cent had more than one. This means that AARs do not, as intended, provide sufficient initial or progress information to allow for the tracking of children's development across seven dimensions' (Department of Health 2001c: 4). Francis (2002) provides limited information on the implementation of the LAC system in Scotland.

2 This instructive contribution was made at a DoH conference held, in London, on 1 July 1997. Subsequently it was circulated to all local authorities implementing the system.

3 Readers are directed to the excellent critical discussions on 'evidence-based' policy and practice and related themes in Newman (2001: 69–72), Taylor and White (2001), Webb (2001) and Sanderson (2002). Specifically in relation to the SCIE, it has been observed that it 'gives a rather listless impression' (see the editorial 'Much still to improve', *Community Care*, 3–9 October 2002: 5).

4 'Working together' to protect children?

1 During the second Blair administration we began to see a broadening out of the policing role into other related spheres of the welfare state, with plans to locate police officers in schools ('Police to be based in schools blighted by truancy', *The*

Guardian, 30 April 2002; see also 'Police officers will have a positive impact on school communities', *Youth Justice Board News*, December 2002: 6).

2 The empirical work took the form of 'semi-structured interviews' and an interviewing schedule was used. I was free, however, to seek clarification and elaboration of the answers given (see also May 1993: ch. 6). This schedule, not seen by the respondent prior to the interviews, focused on four specific areas concerned with child protection: the job of a police officer/social worker; 'working together'; child abuse; criminal justice and social policy. In this chapter, however, the focus will largely be on the first two thematic dimensions. In total, twenty-one respondents took part in the research activity; seven respondents in each practice location; fourteen police officers and seven social workers. I made contemporaneous notes of the respondents' comments and remarks in Whiteley. A cassette tape recorder was taken along to the sessions in the unit, but only the Detective Sergeant (DS) was prepared to allow the interview to be taped. Similarly, in Romley no tape-recording of police officers responses took place, yet here the responses of the social workers sharing the unit were recorded. In Killeen all the respondents were prepared to be tape-recorded. Clearly, advantages and disadvantages are associated with audio-taping. Taping provides greater confidence, perhaps, that a response has been accurately transcribed, but it may also serve to constrain a respondent.

By virtue of being employed – at that time – as a social worker, I was, of course, likely to have been perceived in a particular way by both social workers and police officers from the outset. Thus, with the social workers, I was situated within a specific professional discourse, their own. With the police officers, however, I may have been seen as, in some way, partisan. Perceptions were also likely to have been rendered a good deal more complex, of course, because of issues of 'race' and gender in that a white male police officer, for example, might be more likely to *connect* with a white male researcher than, say, a black female researcher. This point is relevant, but should not, perhaps, be over-emphasised in that it is not being argued that *real* or *authentic* communication can take place only between individuals whose formation is a consequence of where they are situated as 'raced' and gendered subjects. It is, however, to observe that a power relation is present in interview exercises and that interviews do not, of course, take place in a social vacuum (see Kvale 1996). Finally, it should also be observed that social workers and police officers are occupational groups each with their own specific discourse of 'interviewing' and each regards the interviewing (of 'clients', 'suspects' and 'witnesses') as an expertise which they possess.

3 In a submission to the Climbié inquiry, the Commissioner of the Metropolitan Police referred to social services as the '*so-called* "lead" agency'.

4 In this context see Gillen (2002b); also the remarks of Leroy Logan, chair of the London Black Police Association, in 'Police "were racist" in Climbié case', *The Guardian*, 30 April 2002.

PART II THINGS CAN ONLY GET BETTER?

1 Somewhat belatedly, in a less publicised speech two months later, the Prime Minister praised social workers, 'the unsung heroes of the public services', who were a 'force for good in our country'. These comments were made at a reception at No. 10 Downing Street (Department of Health 2002c).

2 This crisis in social work is not confined to the United Kingdom. Similar problems are detectable in the Republic of Ireland (see 'Social workers go on strike', *The Sunday Tribune*, 26 May 2002).

5 Social work and the Third Way

1 *The Child's World: Assessing Children in Need – Reader* (Department of Health 2000b) has also been published as Howarth (ed.) (2001).
2 It could be argued that alongside the renewed valorisation of work within the national territory has been a new emphasis on Britain's international role. More specifically, elements associated with New Labour's 'project' are, in the early twenty-first century, prepared to see Britain undertake a 'new kind of imperialism' within the 'new world order'. Historically, of course, government concerns about the working population being 'fit' for labour *and* for military service have often been enmeshed (Cooper 2002; see also the editorial 'Imperial delusions', *The Guardian*, 29 March 2002).
3 Pierre Bourdieu (2001) and David Harvey (2002) provide two of the most compelling critiques of this dominant understanding of 'globalisation'. Chantal Mouffe (2000: 119) has argued that 'the mantra of globalisation is invoked to justify the *status quo* and reinforce the power of big transnational corporations'. Stephen Webb (2002) has furnished a critique of shallow notions about 'global' social work.
4 Although not a key issue for this particular book it is also interesting to observe how, with the privatisation of social services by state and municipal governments in the United States, the 'defence industry' is profiting from running these programmes. Perhaps the best example is Lockheed Martin, which produces the F-16 fighter jet. It has now become a leading provider of Welfare, having been awarded contracts to run 'Welfare to Work' programmes in a number of states (see also Harris 2002). Unions such as the American Federation of Government Employees (AFGE) have opposed this development.
5 It is acknowledged that Laventi Pavolovich Beria (1899–1953), the head of the NKVD (the Commissariat for Internal Affairs) and 'spymaster' in Stalin's Soviet Union played no role in the formulation of any of the materials associated with the Framework.

6 An 'eye-catching initiative'

1 During phase two of the Climbié inquiry it was also suggested that the new National Adoption Register could be adapted, or copied, to create a national database of children in need of protection (see 'Data sharing could aid information sharing', *Community Care*, 21–27 March 2002: 10 11).
2 See also the remarks of Tim Newburn (2002: 176–7) on New Labour and the image and impression of 'toughness'. The emergence of a new, 'tougher' approach on child welfare can, perhaps, be seen in the so-called 'care proceedings explosion' (Beckett 2001). In terms of children 'looked after' on a compulsory *and* voluntary basis, the number rose from 49,000 in 1994 to 58,100 in 2000. This is a rise of 13 per cent in six years (see ADSS 2002a: 2).

7 Viewing the world through a monochrome lens

1 Social work's ethical base is, of course, rooted in Kantian ethics yet, as Paul Gilroy (2000: 60) has argued, it is rarely acknowledged that 'Kant's democratic hopes and dreams simply did not encompass black humanity'.
2 The term *diaspora* is 'loose in the world' (Clifford in Gray 2000: 168) and diasporas 'must be seen as a product and constituent of international capitalism' (Walter 2001: 8). At its most basic, however, diaspora simply refers to the dispersion or migration of communities. However, as Stuart Hall (1990: 35) has

argued, 'Diaspora does not refer us to those scattered tribes whose identity can only be secured in relation to some sacred homeland . . . the diaspora experience as I intend it here is defined, not by the essence of purity, but by the recognition of a necessary heterogeneity and diversity; by a conception of "identity" which lives by and through, not despite difference; by hybridity. Diaspora identities are those which are constantly producing and reproducing themselves anew, through transformation and difference.'

3 Following the O'Leary judgement of August 2000, Irish Travellers are considered as an ethnic group under the terms of the Race Relations Act 1976.

4 Changes introduced in the 2001 census were, as Hickman *et al.* (2001: 1) observe, a 'significant development, which acknowledges that Irish identities are not simply confined to a migrant generation'. However, unlike in North America and Australia, the 'Irish' category used in the 2001 census was singular rather than mixed or multiple-choice. That is to say, in England and Wales the named 'white' ethnic categories were 'British' and 'Irish', without provision for a 'mixed' category (Walter *et al.* 2002: 31). This fails, therefore, to account for the large proportion of children and young people who may see themselves as having mixed or hybrid identities. Equally important, with the 'children in need' data, there is no indication that children and young people *themselves* were involved in any of the processes leading to national or ethnic identification.

5 This conclusion is drawn from some of the findings which are emerging from a survey of Social Services Departments' responses to Irish children and families in England and Wales which I undertook at the suggestion of the All-party Irish in Britain parliamentary group of MPs in Parliament.

8 Social work with children and families in a world of 'emergent new professionals'

1 Connexions will provide a service for young people with learning difficulties and disabilities until they reach twenty-five years of age.

2 Importantly, however, business plans and checklists will restrain these qualities. The former have already been criticised for focusing too much on young people's academic attainment and employability (see Winchester 2001b). Targets set for pilot programmes, for example, specified increases in the number and grades of qualification which needed to be achieved.

3 Holden Caulfield is the central character in *The Catcher in the Rye* a novel by J. D. Salinger published, in the United States, in 1951. Colley and Hodkinson (2001: 39) have commented on the 'metaphors of descent and fall' in the social exclusion literature. They usefully observe how this can be interpreted as evoking 'Christian connotations of the biblical "Fall" and "original sin"'.

4 'Social Work. It's all about people' was one of the key phrases chosen to 'market' social work training during the recruitment drive in 2001/2. The new social work degree course will be referred to in Chapter 9.

5 Personal advisers will, we are informed, be drawn from 'a range of backgrounds including the Careers Service, Youth Service, Social Services, teachers and YOTs, as well as the voluntary and community sectors' (DfEE 2000a: 45). They may also be retired police officers ('The right Connexions', *Youth Justice Board News* 4, June 2000: 7).

6 In September 2002 it was announced that, from September 2003, social work students would 'benefit from a new bursary scheme worth at least an average of £3,000 per year' (Department of Health 2002f). This will be approximately half the amount provided to those students who are training to become teachers.

On average newly qualified social workers earn £18,000–£20,000 per year (ADSS 2002b: 11).

9 Conclusion

1 In this context, see also Irving and Young (2002) on the utility for social work of some of the ideas of the literary and cultural theorist and philosopher Mikhail Bakhtin.

2 Bauman (2000c: 216) connects developments in the field of criminal justice with developments in the 'world of global finance'. Now, he argues, 'state governments are allotted the role of little more than oversized police precincts; the quality of the policeman on the beat, efficiency displayed in sweeping the streets of beggars, pesterers and pilferers, and the tightness of the jail walls loom large among the factors affecting investors' confidence and so are among the items calculated when the decisions to invest or cut the losses and run are made. To excel in the job of precinct policeman is the best (perhaps the only) thing state governments may do to cajole the nomadic capital into investing in its subjects' welfare.'

Garland (2001), Ladipo (2001) and Wacquant (2002) – amongst others – have commented on the increasing use of incarceration in Western societies (see also 'Cash battle as jails fill up', *The Guardian*, 13 July 2002). In terms of social work in Britain, this trend is reflected in the area of youth justice (see Walsh 2002; Hammond 2002; Jerrom 2002b; Neustatter 2002). The UK now imprisons more children than any other country in Europe, except Germany. Moreover, since 1990 twenty-two children have killed themselves in prison (Howard League 2002b).

Perhaps two 'stories' featured on BBC News are also illustrative of the centrality of crime surveillance, children and young people in the early twenty-first century: 'Schools in fingerprint row', 22 July 2002, http://news.bbc.uk/1/hi/education/2144188.stm; 'Scientists discover "crime gene"', 2 August 2002, http://news.bbc.co.uk/1/hi/health/2165715.stm. See also the consultation paper on so-called 'entitlement cards' (Home Office 2002b), particularly those sections concerned with the recording of biometric information as part of the card scheme. Lyon (2001b) has made a number of telling observations on surveillance after the events of 11 September 2001.

3 On account of the Victoria Climbié case and the manifest failure to gather and collate information, there is understandable emphasis on the need to trawl for and accumulate information in the context of child protection activity.

4 Additionally, Article 8, which seeks to protect 'the right to a private and family life', is undermined by a key subclause. Article 8 (2) states: 'There should be no interference by a public authority with the exercise of this right except such as is in accordance with the law and is necessary in a *democratic society* in the interests of *national security*, public safety *or the economic well-being of the country*, for *the prevention of disorder or crime*, for the protection of health *or morals*, or for the protection of the rights and freedoms of others' (emphases added).

BIBLIOGRAPHY

Adams, C. and Horrocks, C. (1999) 'The location of child protection in relation to the current emphasis on core policing' in Violence against Children Study Group, *Children, Child Abuse and Child Protection*, Chichester: Wiley.

Adcock, M. (2000) 'The Core Assessment process – How to synthesise information and make judgements' in Department of Health, *The Child's World: Assessing Children in Need – Reader*, London: Department of Health.

Adcock, M. and White, R. (1985) *Good Enough Parenting*, London: BAAF.

Ainsley, P., Barnes, T. and Momen, A. (2002) 'Making Connexions: a case study in contemporary social policy', *Critical Social Policy* 22 (2): 376–89.

Alcock, P. (1998) 'Bringing Britain together?' *Community Care*, 26 November–2 December: 18–25.

Alderson, J. (1979) *Policing Freedom*, Plymouth: Macdonald & Evans.

Aldgate, J. (2002) 'Evolution not revolution: family support services and the Children Act 1989' in H. Ward and W. Rose (eds) *Approaches to Needs Assessment in Children's Services*, London: Jessica Kingsley.

Aldgate, J. and Statham, J. (2001) *The Children Act Now: Messages from Research*, London: Stationery Office.

Aldgate, J., Heath, A., Colton, M. and Simm, M. (1993) 'Social work and the education of children in foster care', *Adoption and Fostering* 17 (3): 25–35.

Alexander, C. and Alleyne, B. (2002) 'Framing difference: racial and ethnic studies in twenty-first-century Britain', *Ethnic and Racial Studies* 25 (4): 541–51.

Alibhai-Brown, Y. (1999) 'Whose nature to nurture?' *Community Care*, 1–7 July: 18.

Alibhai-Brown, Y. (2000) 'Muddled leaders and the future of British national identity', *Political Quarterly* 71 (1): 26–31.

Althusser, L. A. (1971) *Lenin and Philosophy and other Essays*, London: New Left Books.

Ansell, S. (2001) 'Connexions and post-16 PSHE: a viable option?' *Youth and Policy* 71: 77–90.

Anthias, F. (1999) 'Institutional racism, power and accountability', *Sociological Research Online* 4 (1), URL (consulted June 1999) http://www.socresonline.org.uk/4/lawrence/anthias.html.

Anthias, F. and Yuval-Davis, N. (1993) *Racialised Boundaries*, London: Routledge.

Archard, D. (1993) *Children, Rights and Childhood*, London: Routledge.

Arkin, A. (2001) 'Blood on the production line', *Public Finance* 16: 24–6.

Arrowsmith, A. (1999) 'Debating diasporic identity: nostalgia, (post)nationalism, "critical traditionalism" ', *Irish Studies Review* 7 (2): 173–83.

Association of Directors of Social Services (2002a) *Tomorrow's Children: a Discussion Paper on UK Child Care Services in the Coming Decade*, London: Association of Directors of Social Services.

Association of Directors of Social Services (2002b) 'Directors reject separate agency as solution to child protection dilemmas', press release, 20 March.

Atherton, C. (1999) 'Towards Evidence Based Services for Children and Families', ESRC-funded 'Theorising Social Work Research' seminar, 20 September, http://www.nisw.org.uk/tswr/atherton.html.

Atkinson, R. (2000) 'Narratives of policy: the construction of urban problems and urban policy in the official discourse of British government 1968–1998', *Critical Social Policy* 20 (2): 211–32.

Audit Commission (1994) *Seen but not Heard: Co-ordinating Community Child Health and Social Services for Children in Need*, London: HMSO.

Back, L., Keith, M., Khan, A., Shukra, K. and Solomos, J. (2002) 'New Labour's white heart: politics, multiculturalism and the return of assimilation', *Political Quarterly* 73 (4): 445–55.

Bailey, R. and Williams, B. (2001) 'No soft option', *Community Care*, 11–17 January: 24–6.

Bain, P., Watson, A., Mulvey, G., Taylor, P. and Gall, G. (2002) 'Taylorism, targets and the pursuit of quantity and quality by call centre management', *New Technology, Work and Employment* 17 (3): 170–86.

Baldry, S. and Kemmis, J. (1998) 'The quality of child care in one local authority: a user study', *Adoption and Fostering* 22 (3): 34–42.

Ball, C. (2001) 'The White Paper *Adoption: a New Approach:* a curate's egg?' *Adoption and Fostering* 25 (1): 6–13.

Ball, S. (2001) 'Performativities and fabrications in the education economy' in D. Gleason and C. Husband (eds) *The Performing School*, London: Taylor & Francis.

Baran, A. and Pannor, R. (1990) 'Open adoption' in D. M. Brodzinsky and M. D. Schechter (eds) *The Psychology of Adoption*. Oxford: Oxford University Press.

Barn R., Sinclair R. and Ferdinand, D. (1997) *Acting on Principle: an Examination of Race and Ethnicity in Social Services Provision for Children and Families*, London: British Agencies for Adoption and Fostering.

Barnes, J. (2002) 'Reform of Social Work Education and Training', http://www.doh.gov.uk/swqualification/focusgroup.pdf.

Bar-on, A. (1999) 'Social work and the "missionary zeal to whip the heathen along the path of righteousness" ', *British Journal of Social Work* 29: 5–26.

Barry, M. and Hallett, C. (eds) (1998) *Social Exclusion and Social Work: Issues of Theory, Policy and Practice*, Lyme Regis: Russell House.

Bauman, Z. (1998) *Work, Consumerism and the New Poor*, Buckingham: Open University Press.

Bauman, Z. (1999) *Globalization: the Human Consequences*, Cambridge: Polity Press.

Bauman, Z. (2000a) 'Am I my brother's keeper?' *European Journal of Social Work* 3 (1): 5–11.

Bauman, Z. (2000b) 'On writing: on writing sociology', *Theory, Culture and Society* 17 (1): 79–90.

Bauman, Z. (2000c) 'Social issues of law and order', *British Journal of Criminology* 40: 205–21.

Bebbington, A. and Miles, J. (1989) 'The background of children who enter local authority care', *British Journal of Social Work* 19: 349–69.

Beck, U. (1994) 'The reinvention of politics: towards a theory of reflexive modernization' in U. Beck, A. Giddens and S. Lash, *Reflexive Modernization*, Cambridge: Cambridge University Press.

Beck, U. (1998) *The Risk Society*, 6th edn, London: Sage.

Becker, S. (1997) *Responding to Poverty: the Politics of Cash and Care*, Harlow: Longman.

Beckett, C. (2001) 'The great care proceedings explosion', *British Journal of Social Work* 31: 493–501.

Beder, S. (2000) *Selling the Work Ethic*, London: Zed Books.

Beek, M. (1994) 'The reality of face-to-face contact after adoption', *Adoption and Fostering* 18 (2): 39–44.

Bell, M. (1998/9) 'The Looking after Children materials: a critical analysis of their use in practice', *Adoption and Fostering* 22 (4): 15–24.

Bell, S. (1988) *When Salem came to the Boro*, London: Pan Books.

Bell, V. (1993) 'Governing childhood: neo-liberalism and the law', *Economy and Society* 22 (3): 390–406.

Bennett, T. (1998) *Culture: a Reformer's Science*, London: Sage.

Beresford, P. and Evans, C. (1999) 'Research note: research and empowerment', *British Journal of Social Work* 29: 671–7.

Berry, M. (2001) *A Sense of Purpose: Care Leavers' Views and Experiences of Growing up*, Edinburgh: Save the Children in Scotland.

Biehal, N., Clayden, J., Stein, M. and Wade, J. (1995) *Moving on: Young People and Leaving Care Schemes*, London: HMSO.

Birkett, D. (2002) 'The instant mums' club', *Guardian G2*, 24 June: 10–11.

Birlson, P. (1981) 'The validity of depressive disorder in childhood and the development of a self-rating scale: a research report', *Journal of Child Psychology and Psychiatry* 22: 73–88.

Blaikie, N. (1993) *Approaches to Social Inquiry*, Cambridge: Polity Press.

Blair, T. (1999) 'Beveridge revisited: a welfare state for the twenty-first century' in R. Walker (ed.) *Ending Child Poverty: Popular Welfare in the Twenty-first Century?* Bristol: Policy Press.

Blair, T. (2000) 'Foreword' in Department for Education and Employment, *Connexions: the Best Start in Life for every Young Person*, Nottingham: DfEE.

Blaug, R. (1995) 'Distortion of the face-to-face: communicative reason and social work practice', *British Journal of Social Work* 25: 423–39.

Bloomfield, B. (2001) 'In the right place at the right time: electronic tagging and problems of social order/disorder', *Sociological Review* 49 (2): 174–202.

Bonnett, A. (2000) *White Identities*, Harlow: Prentice Hall.

Bosanquet, B. (ed.) (1895) *Aspects of the Social Problem*, London: Macmillan.

Bouchier P., Lambert, L. and Triseliotis, J. (1991) *Parting with a Child for Adoption: the Mother's Perspective.* London: BAAF

Bourdieu, P. (1991) *Language and Symbolic Power*, Cambridge: Polity Press.

Bourdieu, P. (2001) *Acts of Resistance: Against the Myths of our Time*, Cambridge: Polity Press.

Bowles, S. (1999) 'Social capital and community governance', *Focus* 20 (3): 6–11.

Bowring, F. (2000) 'Social exclusion: limitations of the debate', *Critical Social Policy* 20 (3): 307–31.

Boyle, M. (2001) 'Towards a (re)theorisation of the historical geography of nationalisms in diasporas: the Irish diaspora as an exemplar', *International Journal of Population Studies* 7: 429–44.

Bracken, P. J. and O'Sullivan, P. (2001) 'The invisibility of Irish migrants in British health records', *Irish Studies Review* 9 (1): 41–53.

Bradshaw, J. and Holmes, H. (1989) *Living on the Edge: a Study of the Living Standards of Families on Benefit in Tyne and Wear*, London: Tyneside Child Poverty Action Group.

Brah, A. (1992) 'Difference, diversity and differentiation' in J. Donald and A. Rattansi (eds) *'Race', Culture and Difference*, London: Sage.

Brandon, M., Schofield, G., Trinder, L. with Stone, N. (1998) *Social Work with Children*, London: Macmillan.

British Association of Social Workers (1996) *A Code of Ethics for Social Work*, Birmingham: BASW.

Broad, B. (ed.) (1999a) *The Politics of Social Work Research and Evaluation*, Birmingham: Venture.

Broad, B. (1999b) 'Peer research: involving young people leaving care as peer researchers – lessons learnt', *Theorising Social Research* seminar, 20 September, http://www.nisw.org.uk/tswr/broad.html.

Brodzinsky, A. B. (1990) 'Surrendering an infant for adoption: the birthmother experience' in D. M. Brodzinsky and M. D. Schechter (eds) *The Psychology of Adoption*, Oxford: Oxford University Press.

Brooks, D., Barth, B. P., Bussiere, A. and Patterson, G. (1999) 'Adoption and race: implementing the Multi-ethnic Placement Act and interethnic adoption provisions', *Social Work* 44 (2): 167–79.

Brown, L. and Fuller, C. (1991a) *Joint Police/Social Work Investigation in Child Protection*, Stirling: University of Stirling.

Brown, L. and Fuller, C. (1991b) 'Central Scotland's joint police and social work initiative in child abuse: an evaluation', *Children and Society* 5 (3): 232–40.

Brown, L. and Heinensohn, F. (2000) *Gender and Policing*, London: Macmillan.

Bruegel, I. (2000) 'No more jobs for the boys? Gender and class in the restructuring of the British economy', *Capital and Class* 71: 79–102.

Bullock, R. (1995) 'Change in organisations: likely problems in implementing Looking after Children' in H. Ward (ed.) *Looking after Children: Research into Practice*, London: HMSO.

Burchill, J. (2002) 'Let's all have a flutter', *Guardian Magazine*, 29 June: 5.

Burman, E. (1994) *Deconstructing Developmental Psychology*, London: Routledge.

Burrows, G. (2001) 'Unison vows to fight care trusts amid fears of "medical muddle"', *Community Care*, 21–27 June: 4–5.

159

Busteed. M. (1999) 'Little Islands of Erin: Irish settlement and identity in mid-nineteenth-century Manchester', *Immigrants and Minorities* 18 (2–3): 94–128.

Butler, I. and Drakeford, M. (2001) 'Which Blair Project? Communitarianism, social authoritarianism and social work', *Journal of Social Work* 1 (1): 7–19.

Butler, I. and Payne, H. (1997) 'The health of children looked after by the local authority', *Adoption and Fostering* 21 (2): 28–36.

Byrne, D. (1999) *Social Exclusion*, Buckingham: Open University Press.

Cabinet Office (2000) *The Prime Minister's Review of Adoption: a Performance and Innovation Unit Report*, London: Stationery Office.

Calder, A. (2000) 'Financial support for care leavers', *Poverty* 106: 106–14.

Cameron, C., Mooney, A. and Moss, P. (2002) 'The child care work force: current conditions and future directions', *Critical Social Policy* 22 (4): 572–96.

Campbell, B. (1988) *Unofficial Secrets*, London: Virago.

Campbell, B. (1993) *Goliath*, London: Methuen.

Campbell, B. (1995a) 'Little Beirut', *Guardian*: 1 July.

Campbell, B. (1995b) 'Old fogeys and angry young men: a critique of communitarianism', *Soundings* 1: 47–65.

Campbell, B. (1996) 'Muddled waters', *Community Care*, 10–16 October: 17.

Campbell, B. (1997) 'Wherever they may be', *Community Care*, 10–16 April: 19.

Campbell, B. (2000) 'A mother should know', *Community Care*, 1–7 June 2000: 10.

Campbell, L. H., Silverman, P. R. and Patti, P. B. (1991) 'Reunions between adoptees and birth parents: the adoptees' experience', *Social Work* 36 (4): 329–36.

Campbell, S. (1999) 'Beyond the "plastic paddy": a re-examination of the second generation Irish in England', *Immigrants and Minorities* 18 (2–3): 268–89.

Canny, A., Green, A. E. and Maguire, M. (2001) 'Keeping track of vulnerable young people: a policy agenda', *Youth and Policy* 72: 16–35.

Cantwell, B. (2000) 'The welfare checklist and the assessment of the needs of children', *Family Law*, December: 921–5.

Carter, J. (ed.) (1998) *Postmodernism and the Fragmentation of Welfare*, London: Routledge.

Casey, C. (1995) *Work, Self and Society*, London: Routledge.

Castles, S. and Davidson, A. (2000) *Citizenship and Migration*, London: Macmillan.

Central Council for Education and Training in Social Work (1995) *Assuring Quality in the Diploma in Social Work, 1, Rules and Requirements for the Diploma in Social Work*, London: CCETSW.

Central Council for Education and Training in Social Work (1997) *Using the Looking after Children Materials in Social Work Education and Training*, London: CCETSW.

Chambers, L. (1998) 'Making it alone: a study of the care experiences of young black people', *Childright* 145: 7–19.

Channer, Y. and Parton, N. (1990) 'Racism, cultural relativism and child protection' in Violence against Children Study Group, *Taking Child Abuse Seriously*, London: Unwin Hyman.

Cheetham, J. (1972) *Social Work with Immigrants*, London: Routledge.

Chiapello, E. and Fairclough, N. (2002) 'Understanding the new management ideology: a transdisciplinary contribution from critical discourse analysis and a new sociology of capitalism', *Discourse and Society* 13 (2): 185–208.

Clapton, G. (1997) 'Birth fathers, the adoption process and fatherhood', *Adoption and Fostering* 21 (1): 29 37.

Clark, P. (2002) 'Smaller, but better formed?' *Community Care*, 7–13 February: 38–40.

Clark, S. (1993) 'Adoption decision gets DoH approval', *Community Care*, 16 September: 3.

Clarke, J. and Newman, J. (1997) *The Managerial State*, London: Sage.

Cleaver, H. (2000) 'When parents' issues influence their ability to respond to children's needs' in Department of Health, *The Child's World: Assessing Children in Need – Reader*, London: Department of Health.

Cleaver, H. and Freeman, P. (1995) *Parental Perspectives in Cases of Suspected Child Abuse*, London: HMSO.

Cleaver, H., Unell, I. and Aldgate, J. (1999) *Children's Needs – Parenting Capacity*, London: HMSO.

Clinton, President Bill (2000) State of the Union address, 27 January, http://www.washingtonpost.com/wp-srv/politics/special/states/docs/sou00.htm.

Cochran, M. M. and Brassard, J. A. (1979) 'Child development and personal social networks', *Child Development* 50: 601–16.

Cohen, P. (1994) 'Yesterday's words, tomorrow's world: from the racialisation of adoption to the politics of difference' in I. Gaber and J. Aldridge (eds) *In the Best Interests of the Child: Culture, Identity and Transracial Adoption*, London: Free Association.

Cohen, R. (1994) *Frontiers of Identity: the British and Others*, London: Longman.

Cohen, R. and Tarpey, M. (1988) *Single Payments: the Disappearing Safety Net*, London: Child Poverty Action Group.

Cohen, S. (1979) 'The punitive city: notes on the dispersal of social control', *Contemporary Crises* 3: 339–63.

Cohen, S. (1985) *Visions of Social Control*, Cambridge: Polity Press.

Cohen, S. (2002) 'The local state of immigration controls', *Critical Social Policy* 22 (3): 518–44.

Coleman, J. S. (1988) 'Social capital in the creation of human capital', *American Journal of Sociology* 94 (supplement): 95–120.

Colley, H. (2001) 'An ABC of mentors' talk about disaffected youth: alternative lifestyles, benefit dependency or complete dunces', *Youth and Policy* 72: 1–16.

Colley, H. and Hodkinson, P. (2001) 'Problems with *Bridging the Gap*: the reversal of structure and agency in addressing social exclusion', *Critical Social Policy* 21 (3): 335–59.

Colton, M. (1989) 'Foster and residential children's perceptions of their social environments', *British Journal of Social Work* 19: 217–35.

Commission on Social Justice (1994) *Social Justice: Strategies for National Renewal*, London: Vintage.

Conroy S., Fielding, N. G. and Tunstill, J. (1990) *Investigating Child Sexual Abuse: the Study of a Joint Initiative*, London: Police Foundation.

Cooper, R. (2002) 'Why we still need empires', *Observer*, 7 April.

Coote, A. (2002) 'Star rating is right', *Community Care*, 31 January 6 February: 20.

Coppock, V. (1996) 'Mad, bad or misunderstood?' *Youth and Policy* 53: 53–66.

Corlyn, J. and McGuire, C. (1998) *Young Parents in Public Care*, London: National Children's Bureau.

Corrick, H., Jones, J. and Ward, H. (1995) *Looking after Children: Good Parenting, Good Outcomes: Management and Implementation Guide*, London: HMSO.

Cotson, D., Friend, J., Hollins, S. and James, H. (2000) 'Implementing the framework for the assessment of children in need and their families when the parent has learning difficulties' in Department of Health, *The Child's World: Assessing Children in Need – Reader*, London: Department of Health.

Coward, R. (1997) 'Our children's absolute right to be bone idle', *Guardian*, 9 June.

Craig, G. (ed.) (1989) *Your Flexible Friend: Voluntary Organisations, Claimants and the Social Fund*, London: Child Poverty Action Group.

Crnic, K. A. and Greenberg, M. T. (1990) 'Minor parenting stresses with young children', *Child Development* 61: 1628–37.

Crowther, C. (2000) 'Thinking about the underclass: towards a political economy of policing', *Theoretical Criminology* 4 (2): 149–67.

Dale, P., Davies, M., Morrison, T. and Waters, J. (1986) *Dangerous Families*, London: Tavistock.

Dalrymple, J. and Burke, B. (1995) *Anti-oppressive Practice*, Buckingham: Open University Press.

Dandeker, C. (1990) *Surveillance, Power and Modernity*, Cambridge: Polity Press.

Darling, A. (1999) 'Work is the way off Welfare', *Guardian*, 16 June.

Davies, G., Marshall, E. and Robertson, N. (1998) *Child Abuse: Training Investigating Officers*, London: Home Office.

Deacon, A. (2000) 'Learning from the US? The influence of American ideas upon "New Labour" thinking on Welfare reform', *Policy and Politics* 28 (1): 5–18.

Deacon, A. (2002) 'Echoes of Sir Keith? New Labour and the cycle of disadvantage', *Benefits* 10 (3): 179–85.

Deacon, A. and Mann, K. (1999) 'Agency, modernity and social policy', *Journal of Social Policy* 28: 413–35.

Dean, H. (1992) 'Poverty discourse and the disempowerment of the poor', *Critical Social Policy* 35: 79–89.

Dean, M. (1999) *Governmentality: Power and Rule in Modern Society*, London: Sage.

Delaney, E. (1999) 'Almost a class of helots in an alien land: the British state and Irish immigration 1921–1945', *Immigrants and Minorities* 18 (2–3): 25–45.

Delanty, G. (1997) *Social Science: Beyond Constructivism and Realism*, Buckingham: Open University Press.

Dendy, H. (1895) 'The industrial residuum' in B. Bosanquet (ed.) *Aspects of the Social Problem*, London: Macmillan.

Denham, A. and Garnett, M. (2002) 'From the "cycle of enrichment" to the "cycle of deprivation": Sir Keith Joseph, "problem families" and the transmission of disadvantage', *Benefits* 10 (3): 193–9.

Dennis, N. (1993) *Rising Crime and the Dismembered Family*, London: Institute of Economic Affairs Health and Welfare Unit.

Dennis, N. and Erdos, G. (1993) *Fathers without Families*, London: IEA Health and Welfare Unit.

Department for Education and Employment (1999) *Learning to Succeed: a new Framework for post-16 Learning*, Cm 4392, London: Stationery Office.

Department for Education and Employment (2000a) *Connexions: the Best Start in Life for every Young Person*, Nottingham: DfEE.

Department for Education and Employment (2000b) *The Connexions Service: Professional Framework for Personal Advisers – Proposals for Consultation*, Nottingham: DfEE.

Department for Education and Employment (2000c) *The Connexions Service: Prospectus and Specification*, Nottingham: DfEE.

Department for Education and Employment (2001a) 'Blair sets out next phase of New Deal in government drive to full employment', press notice, 14 March.

Department for Education and Employment (2001b) 'Nissan says New Deal is good for business', press notice, 9 April.

Department for Education and Employment (2001c) *Get Involved . . . to make a Difference*, Nottingham: DfEE.

Department for Education and Employment (2001d) 'Job seekers and parents get boost to improve basic skills', press notice, 30 April.

Department for Education and Employment (2001e) *The Active Involvement of Young People in the Connexions Service: Managers' Guide and Practitioners' Guide*, Nottingham: DfEE.

Department of Health (1988) *Protecting Children: a Guide for Social Workers undertaking a Comprehensive Assessment*, London: HMSO.

Department of Health (1995a) *Child Protection: Messages from the Research*, London: HMSO.

Department of Health (1995b) *Looking after Children: Good Parenting, Good Outcomes Training Guide*, London: HMSO.

Department of Health (1995c) *The Challenge of Partnership in Child Protection*, London: HMSO.

Department of Health (1996) *Children Looked after by Local Authorities, Year ending 31 March 1995: England*, London: Government Statistical Service.

Department of Health (1998a) *Objectives for Social Services for Children*, London: HMSO.

Department of Health (1998b) *Quality Protects: Framework for Action*, London: HMSO.

Department of Health (1998c) *Statistical Bulletin: Children looked after in England, 1997/98*, London: HMSO.

Department of Health (1998d) *Modernising Social Services*, London: HMSO.

Department of Health (1998e) *Someone else's Children*, London: HMSO.

Department of Health (1998f) *Adoption: Achieving the Right Balance*, LAC (98) 20, London: HMSO.

Department of Health (1999a) *Framework for the Assessment of Children in Need and their Families: Consultation Draft*, London: Department of Health.

Department of Health (1999b) *Adoption Now: Messages from Research*, Chichester: Wiley.

Department of Health (1999c) 'Tide is turning on adoption', press release, 18 October.

Department of Health (2000a) *The Children Act Report, 1995–1999*, London: HMSO.

Department of Health (2000b) *The Child's World: Assessing Children in Need – Reader*, London: Department of Health.

Department of Health (2000c) *Assessing Children in Need and their Families: Practice Guidance*, London: Stationery Office.

Department of Health (2000d) '150 teenage pregnancy co-ordinators appointed to drive campaign to cut teenage pregnancy', press release, 29 February.

Department of Health (2000e) *Adoption: a New Approach*, London: HMSO.

Department of Health (2000f) 'More work needed to overturn barriers to adoption', press release, 10 April.

Department of Health (2000g) 'Prime Minister announces action to overhaul adoption process', press release, 7 July.

Department of Health (2000h) 'Social services for children from ethnic minorities must be improved', press notice, 11 July.

Department of Health (2001a) 'Social worker recruitment drive set to be a success', press notice, 28 December.

Department of Health (2001b) 'Milburn orders inquiry into the death of Victoria Climbié', press notice, 12 January.

Department of Health (2001c) *Integrated Children's System*, Briefing Paper No. 3, London: Department of Health.

Department of Health (2001d) 'New social care institute for excellence will raise standards and tackle inconsistencies', press notice, 25 February.

Department of Health (2001e) 'Combating violence against social care staff: new national plan to protect workers', press notice, 23 January.

Department of Health (2001f) *The Children Act Report 2000*, London: Department of Health.

Department of Health (2001g) *Statistical Bulletin: Personal Social Services Staff of Social Services Departments at 30 September 2000: England*, London: Department of Health.

Department of Health (2002a) 'Social services staffing at 30 September 2001', press release, 25 April.

Department of Health (2002b) 'New social work degree will focus on practical training', press release, 22 May.

Department of Health (2002c) 'Social services praised by Prime Minister', press release, 18 March.

Department of Health (2002d) 'Vulnerable children at forefront of local action plans', press release, 14 May.

Department of Health (2002e) 'Future social services investment depends on radical reform', press release, 13 March.

Department of Health (2002f) 'Funding boost for social work students', press release, 30 September.

Department of Health, Cox, A. and Bentovim, A. (2000) *Framework for the Assessment of Children in Need and their Families: The Family Pack of Questionnaiares and Scales*, London: HMSO.

Department of Health, Department for Education and Employment, Home Office (2000) *Framework for the Assessment of Children in Need and their Families*, London: Stationery Office.

Department of Health, Home Office, Department for Education and Employment (1999) *Working Together to Safeguard Children: a Guide to Inter-agency Working to Safeguard and Promote the Welfare of Children*, London: Stationery Office.

Department of Health, NSPCC, University of Sheffield (2000) *The Child's World: Assessing Children in Need – Trainer Modules*, London: Department of Health.

Department of Health, Welsh Office (1992) *Review of Adoption Law: Report to Ministers of an Inter-departmental Working Party*, London: HMSO.

Department of Health, Welsh Office, Home Office, Lord Chancellor's Department (1993) *Adoption: the Future*, Cm 2288, London: HMSO.

Department of Social Security (1999) *Opportunity for All: Tackling Poverty and Social Exclusion*, http://www.dss.gov.uk/hq/pubs/poverty/main/htm.

Dingwell, R. (1999) 'Risk society: the cult theory of the millennium?' *Social Policy and Administration* 33 (4): 474–91.

Dobson, A. (2002) 'Review offers sweeping agenda to safeguard children treated in Wales', *Community Care*, 14–20 March: 18–20.

Dobson, F. (1998) *Quality Protects: Transforming Children's Services: The Role and Responsibilities of Councillors*, London: Department of Health.

Dominelli, L. (1988) *Anti-racist Social Work*, London: Macmillan.

Dominelli, L. (1998) 'Anti-oppressive practice in context' in R. Adams, L. Dominelli and M. Payne (eds) *Social Work: Themes, Issues and Critical Debates*, London: Macmillan.

Dominelli, L. and Hoogvelt, A. (1996) 'Globalization and the technocratization of social work', *Critical Social Policy* 47: 45–63.

Dominelli, L., Lorenz, W. and Soyden, H. (2001) *Beyond Racial Divides: Ethnicities in Social Work Practice*, Aldershot: Avebury.

Donzelot, J. (1979) *The Policing of Families*, London: Hutchinson.

Dooley, B. (1998) *Black and Green: the Fight for Civil Rights in Northern Ireland and Black America*, London: Pluto Press.

Dowling, M. (1999) 'Social exclusion, inequality and social work', *Social Policy and Administration* 33 (3): 245–61.

Downey, R. (2002) 'Which path?' *Community Care*, 25–31 July: 34–7.

Duncan, W. (1993) 'The Hague Convention on the Protection of Children and co-operation in respect of intercountry adoption', *Adoption and Fostering* 17 (3): 9–14.

Durlauf, S. N. (1999) 'The case against social capital', *Focus* 20 (3): 1–6.

Dutt, R. and Phillips, M. (2000) 'Assessing black children and their families' in Department of Health, *Assessing Children in Need and their Families: Practice Guidance*, London: Stationery Office.

Dutt, R. and Sanyal, A. (1991) ' "Openness" in adoption or open adoption: a Black perspective', *Adoption and Fostering* 15 (4): 111–15.

Dyer, R. (1997) *White*, London: Routledge.

Early, T. J. (2001) 'Measures for practice with families from a strengths perspective', *Families in Society* 82 (2): 225–33.

Eason, P., Atkins, M. and Dyson, A. (2000) 'Inter-professional collaboration and conceptualisations of practice', *Children and Society* 14: 355–67.

Easthope, A. and McGowan, K. (eds) (1998) *A Critical and Cultural Theory Reader*, Buckingham: Open University Press.

Eden, L., Bowdler, D. and Thorpe, R. (2002) 'Fertile work', *Community Care*, 28 March–3 April: 38–40.

Edge, S. (1995) 'Women are trouble, did you know that, Fergus?' *Feminist Review* 50: 173–86.

Edwards, R. and Usher, R. (1994) 'Disciplining the subject: the power of competence', *Studies in the Education of Adults* 26 (1): 1–15.

Eisenstadt, N. (1998) 'Changing times', *Community Care*, 3–9 September: 16.

Engel, M. (1999) 'My daughter's Big Brother', *Guardian Weekend*, 29 May: 10–18.

Engels, F. (1926) *The Condition of the Working Class in England in 1844*, trans. F. K. Wischnewetzky, London: Allen & Unwin.

Ennew, J. (1994) 'Time for children or time for adults?' in J. Qvortrup (ed.) *Childhood Matters: Social Theory, Practice and Politics*, Aldershot: Avebury.

Etzioni, A. (1995) *The Spirit of the Community: Rights, Responsibilities and the Communitarian Agenda*, London: Fontana.

Etzioni, A. (2001) 'Is bowling together sociologically Lite?' *Contemporary Sociology* 30 (3): 223–5.

Eysenck, H. J. (1971) *Race, Intelligence and Education*, London: Temple Smith.

Fabricant, M. (1985) 'The industrialization of social work practice', *Social Work* 30 (5): 389–96.

Fabricant, M. B. and Burghardt, S. (1992) *The Welfare State Crisis and the Transformation of Social Service Work*, New York: Sharpe.

Fairclough, N. (1999) *Discourse and Social Change*, 6th edn, Cambridge: Polity Press.

Fairclough, N. (2000) *New Labour, New Language?* London: Routledge.

Family Policy Unit (1998) *Supporting Families*, London: Stationery Office.

Fawcett, B. and Featherstone, B. (1998) 'Quality assurance and evaluation in social work in a postmodern era' in J. Carter (ed.) *Postmodernity and the Fragmentation of Welfare*, London: Routledge.

Fawcett, B., Featherstone, B., Fook, J. and Rossiter, A. (eds) (2000) *Practice and Research in Social Work: Postmodern Feminist Perspectives*, London: Routledge.

Feast, J. and Howe, D. (1997) 'Adopted adults who search for background information and contact with birth relatives', *Adoption and Fostering* 21 (2): 8–16.

Fekete, L. (2001) 'The emergence of xeno-racism', *Race and Class* 43 (2): 23–40.

Ferguson, I. and Lavalette, M. (1999) 'Social work, postmodernism, and Marxism', *European Journal of Social Work* 2 (1): 27–40.

Fergusson, R., Pye, D., Esland, G., McLaughlin, E. and Muncie, J. (2000) 'Normalized dislocation and new subjectivities in post-16 markets for education and work', *Critical Social Policy* 64: 28–51.

Findlay, C. (1991) 'Joint police and social work investigations in child abuse: a practice example from Scotland', *Children and Society* 5 (3): 225–31.

Finn, J. L. and Nybell, L. (2001) 'Capitalizing on concern: the making of troubled children and troubling youth in late capitalism', *Childhood* 8 (2): 139–45.

Fitzpatrick, T. (2001) 'New agendas for social policy and criminology: globalization, urbanism and the emerging post-social security state', *Social Policy and Administration* 35 (2): 212–29.

Fitzpatrick, T. (2002) 'In search of welfare democracy', *Social Policy and Society* 1 (1): 11–21.

Fletcher-Campbell, F. (1998) 'Progress or procrastination? The education of young people who are looked after', *Children and Society* 12: 3 11.

Flynn, R. (2000) 'Black carers for white children: shifting the "same race" debate', *Adoption and Fostering* 24 (1): 47–53.

Ford, J. (1991) *Consuming Credit: Debt and Poverty in the UK*, London: Child Poverty Action Group.

Forrest, D. (2000) 'Theorising empowerment thought: illuminating the relationship between ideology and politics in the contemporary era', *Sociological Research Online*, 4 (4), http://www.socresonline.org.uk/4/4/forrest.html.

Forsythe, B. (1995) 'Discrimination in social work', *British Journal of Social Work* 25 (1): 1–17.

Foster, P. and Wilding, P. (2000) 'Whither Welfare professionalism?' *Social Policy and Administration* 34 (2): 143–59.

Foucault, M. (1977) *Discipline and Punish*, Harmondsworth: Penguin.

Fox, N. J. (1993) *Postmodernism, Sociology and Health*, London: Sage.

Fox Harding, L. M. (1991) *Perspectives in Child Care*, London: Longman.

Francis, J. (2002) 'Implementing the "Looking after Children in Scotland" materials: panacea or stepping-stone?' *Social Work Education* 21 (4): 449–61.

Franklin, B. (ed.) (1995) *Children's Rights*, London: Routledge.

Fraser, N. (1989) *Unruly Practices: Power, Discourse and Gender in Contemporary Social Theory*, Cambridge: Polity Press.

Fraser, N. (2000) 'Rethinking recognition', *New Left Review*, May–June: 107–21.

Freeman, M. D. A. (1983) *The Rights and Wrongs of Children*, London: Pinter.

Freely, M. (1999) 'Teaching mothers a lesson', *Guardian*, 29 September.

Froggett, L. and Sapey, B. (1997) 'Communication, culture and social work', *Social Work Education* 16 (1): 41–54.

Fukuyama, F. (1992) *The End of History and the Last Man*. London: Hamish Hamilton.

Fuller, R. and Petch, A. (1995) *Practitioner Research*, Buckingham: Open University Press.

Furlong, A. and Cartmel, F. (1997) *Young People and Social Change: Individualization and Risk in late Modernity*, Buckingham: Open University Press.

Gamble, A., Marsh, D. and Tant, T. (1999) *Marxism and Social Science*, London: Macmillan.

Gardiner, M. A. S. (1991) *Towards a Model for the Implementation and Management of a Joint Sexual Abuse Investigation Scheme between the Police and Social Services*, Hampshire: Hampshire County Council Social Services Department.

Garland, D. (2001) *The Culture of Control: Crime and Social Order in Contemporary Society*, Oxford: Oxford University Press.

Garrett, P. M. (1998) 'Notes from the diaspora: anti-discriminatory social work practice, Irish people and the practice curriculum', *Social Work Education* 17 (4): 435–49.

Garrett, P. M. (2000a) 'The "abnormal flight": the migration and repatriation of Irish unmarried mothers', *Social History* 25 (3): 330–44.

Garrett, P. M. (2000b) 'Responding to Irish "invisibility": anti-discriminatory social work practice and the placement of Irish children in Britain', *Adoption and Fostering* 24 (1): 23–34.

Garrett, P. M. (2000c) 'The hidden history of the PFIs: the repatriation of un-married mothers and their children from England to Ireland in the 1950s and 1960s', *Immigrants and Minorities* 19 (3): 25–44.

Garrett, P. M. (2001) 'Interrogating *Home Alone*: the critical deconstruction of media representations in social work education', *Social Work Education* 20 (6): 643–59.

Garrett, P. M. (2002) 'Social Work and the "just society": diversity, difference and the sequestration of poverty', *Journal of Social Work* 2 (2): 187–210.

Garrett, P. M. (2003a) 'The "daring experiment": the London County Council and the discharge from care of children to Ireland in the 1950s and 1960s', *Journal of Social Policy* 32 (1): 1–18.

Garrett, P. M. (2003b) 'The trouble with Harry: why the "new agenda of life politics" fails to convince', *British Journal of Social Work*, 33 (3): 381–97.

Garrett, P. M. and Sinkkonen, J. (2003) 'Putting children first? A comparison of child adoption policy and practice in Britain and Finland', *European Journal of Social Work* 6 (1): 19–33.

Gibbons, J. (1991) *Fife Child Protection Unit: Report of the research consultancy carried out by the National Institute of Social Work*, London: National Institute of Social Work.

Giddens, A. (1978) 'Positivism and its critics' in T. Bottomore and R. Nisbet (eds) *A History of Sociological Analysis*, London: Heinemann.

Giddens, A. (1989) *Sociology*, Cambridge: Polity Press.

Gillen, S. (2002a) 'Lauren Wright case exposes lack of training for GPs in child protection', *Community Care*, 11–17 April: 18–20.

Gillen, S. (2002b) 'Was race an issue?' *Community Care*, 21–27 February: 30–2.

Gilley, S. (1999) 'Roman Catholicism and the Irish in England', *Immigrants and Minorities* 18 (2–3): 147–68.

Gilroy, P. (1994) 'Foreword' in I. Gaber and J. Aldridge (eds) *In the Best Interests of the Child: Culture, Identity and Transracial Adoption*, London: Free Association.

Gilroy, P. (1998) 'Race ends here', *Ethnic and Racial Studies* 21 (5): 838–48.

Gilroy, P. (2000) *Between Camps: Nations, Cultures and the Allure of Race*, London: Penguin.

Giroux, H. A. (2000) 'Public pedagogy as cultural politics', *Cultural Studies* 14 (2): 341–60.

Glass, N. (1999) 'Sure Start: the development of an early intervention programme in the United Kingdom', *Children and Society* 13: 257–64.

Gledhill, A. (1989) *Who Cares?* London: Centre for Policy Studies.

Goldson, B. (2000) 'Children in need or young offenders? Hardening ideology, organizational change and new challenges for social work with children in trouble', *Child and Family Social Work* 5: 255–65.

Gorman, J. (1993) 'Postmodernism and the conduct of inquiry in social work', *Affilia* 8 (3): 247–65.

Gray, B. (2000) 'Gendering the Irish diaspora: questions of enrichment, hybridization and return', *Women's International Review* 23 (2): 167–85.

Gray, J. (2000) preface in Department of Health, *The Child's World: Assessing Children in Need – Reader*, London: Department of Health.

Gray, J. (2002) 'National policy on the assessment of children in need and their families' in H. Ward and W. Rose (eds) *Approaches to Needs Assessment in Children's Services*, London: Jessica Kingsley.

Graybeal, C. (2001) 'Strengths-based social work assessment: transforming the dominant paradigm', *Families in Society* 82 (2): 233–43.

Green, A. E., Maguire, M. and Canny, A. (2001) *Keeping Track: Mapping and Tracking Vulnerable Young People*, Bristol: Policy Press.

Green, L. (2000) 'Anti-poverty plans lack workers' input', *Community Care*, 22–8 June: 10–11.

Greenslade, L. (1992) 'White skin, white masks: psychological distress among the Irish in Britain' in P. O'Sullivan (ed.) *The Irish in the New Communities*, London: Leicester University Press.

Groothues, C., Beckett, C. and O'Connor, T. (1998/9) 'The outcome of adoptions from Romania', *Adoption and Fostering* 22 (4): 30–41.

Gubruim, J. F., Buckholdt, D. R. and Lynott, R. J. (1989) 'The descriptive tyranny of forms', *Perspectives on Social Problems* 1: 195–214.

Gudmundsdottir, S. (1996) 'The teller, the tale and the one being told: the narrative nature of the research interview', *Curriculum Inquiry* 26 (3). 293–307.

Gupta, A. (2002) 'Sacrificed for targets?' *Community Care*, 25 April–2 May: 42–3.

Habermas, J. (1996) 'Knowledge and human interests: a general perspective' in William Outhwaite (ed.) *The Habermas Reader*, Cambridge: Polity Press.

Haggerty, K. D. and Ericson, R. V. (2000) 'The surveillant assemblage', *British Journal of Sociology* 51 (4): 605–22.

Hall, M. P. (1960) *The Social Services of Modern England*, London: Routledge.

Hall, S. (1990) 'Cultural identity and diaspora' in J. Rutherford (ed.) *Identity: Community, Culture, Difference*, London: Lawrence & Wishart.

Hall, S. (1992a) 'New ethnicities' in J. Donald and A. Rattansi (eds) *'Race', Culture and Difference*, London: Sage.

Hall, S. (1992b) 'Our mongrel selves', *New Statesman and Society*, 19 June: 6–8.

Hall, S. (1993) 'Thatcherism today', *New Statesman and Society*, 26 November: 14–17.

Hall, S. (1998) 'The Great Moving Nowhere Show', *Marxism Today*, November–December: 9–15.

Hall, S. and du Gay, P. (1998) (eds) *Questions of Identity*, 4th edn, London: Sage.

Hall, S. and Jacques, M. (1989) *New Times: the Changing Face of Politics in the 1990s*, London: Lawrence & Wishart.

Hallett, C. (1995) *Interagency Co-ordination in Child Protection*, London: HMSO.

Hallett, C. and Birchall, E. (1992) *Co-ordination and Child Protection: a Review of the Literature*, Edinburgh: HMSO.

Hallett, C. and Stevenson, O. (1980) *Child Abuse: Aspects of Inter-professional Co-operation*, London: Allen & Unwin.

Hammond, D. (2002) 'More children deprived of liberty as Welfare and justice systems collide', *Community Care*, 11–17 July: 18–20.

Handler, J. (2000) 'Reforming/deforming Welfare', *New Left Review* 4: 114–37.

Harding, S. and Balarajan, R. (2001) 'Mortality of third-generation Irish people living in England and Wales: longitudinal study', *British Medical Journal* 322: 466–7.

Harmon, C. (1988) *The Fire Next Time: 1968 and After*, London: Bookmark.

Harris, C. (2001) 'Beyond multiculturalism? Difference, recognition and social justice', *Patterns of Prejudice* 35 (1): 13–35.

Harris, J. (1998) 'Scientific management, bureau-professionalism, new managerialism: the labour process of state social work', *British Journal of Social Work* 28: 839–62.

Harris, J. (2001) 'Information technology and the global ruling class', *Race and Class* 42 (4): 35–56.

Harris, J. (2002) 'The US military in the era of globalisation', *Race and Class* 44 (2): 1–22.

Harris, P. (1999) 'Public welfare and liberal governance' in A. Petersen, I. Barns, J. Dudley, J. and P. Harris (eds) *Poststructuralism, Citizenship and Social Policy*, London: Routledge.

Harris, P. (2002) 'Welfare rewritten: change and interplay in social and economic accounts', *Journal of Social Policy* 31 (3): 377–99.

Harrison, S. (2002) 'New Labour, modernisation and the medical labour process', *Journal of Social Policy* 31 (3): 465–87.

Harvey, D. (1990) *The Condition of Postmodernity*, Oxford: Blackwell.

Harvey, D. (2002) *Spaces of Hope*, Edinburgh: Edinburgh University Press.

Harvie, D. (2000) 'Alienation, class and enclosure in UK universities', *Capital and Class* 71: 103–33.

Hayden, C., Goddard, J., Gorin, S. and Van Der Spek, N. (1999) *State Child Care*, London: Jessica Kingsley.

Hayes, D. (2002) 'Minister rolls out latest phase of strategy to cut teenage pregnancies', *Community Care*, 4–10 July: 10.

Haylett, C. (2001a) 'Illegitimate subjects? Abject white, neoliberal modernisation, and middle-class multiculturalism', *Economy and Planning D: Society and Space* 19: 351–70.

Haylett, C. (2001b) 'Modernisation, welfare and "third way" politics: limits in "thirds"?' *Transactions of the Institute of British Geographers* 26 (1): 43–56.

Heath, A., Colton, M. and Aldgate, J. (1989) 'The educational progress of children in and out of care', *British Journal of Social Work* 19: 447–60.

Hendrick, H. (1990) 'Constructions and reconstructions of British childhood: an interpretative survey, 1800 to the present' in A. James and A. Prout (eds) *Constructing and Reconstructing Childhood: Contemporary Issues in the Sociological Study of Childhood*, London: Falmer.

Hendrick, H. (1994) *Child Welfare: England, 1872–1989*, London: Routledge.

Henricson, C., Coleman, J. and Roker, D. (2000) 'Parenting in the youth justice context', *Howard Journal* 39 (4): 325–38.

Her Majesty's Inspectorate of Constabulary (1999) *Child Protection: What does it mean for the Police Service?* London: Home Office.

Hickman, M. J. (1996) 'Incorporating and denationalizing the Irish in England: the role of the Catholic Church' in P. O'Sullivan (ed.) *Religion and Identity*, London: Leicester University Press.

Hickman, M. J. (1998) 'Reconstructing/deconstructing "race": British political discourses about the Irish in Britain', *Ethnic and Racial Studies* 21 (2): 288–307.

Hickman, M. (2000) 'Binary opposites or unique neighbours? The Irish in multi-ethnic Britain', *Political Quarterly* 71 (1): 50–7.

Hickman, M. J. and Walter, B. (1997) *Discrimination and the Irish Community in Britain*, London: Commission for Racial Equality.

Hickman, M. J, Morgan, S. and Walter, B. (2001) *Second-generation Irish People in Britain*, London: Irish Studies Centre, University of North London.

Hicks, C. and Tite, R. (1998) 'Professional attitudes about the victims of child sexual abuse: implications for collaborative child protection teams', *Child and Family Social Work* 3: 37–48.

Higham, P. (2001) 'Changing practice and an emerging social pedagogue paradigm in England: the role of the personal adviser', *Social Work in Europe* 8 (1): 21–9.

Hill, M. (ed.) (1993) *The Policy Process: a Reader*, Hemel Hempstead: Harvester Wheatsheaf.

Hillyard, P. (1993) *Suspect Community*, London: Pluto.

Hillyard, P. and Percy-Smith, J. (1988) *The Coercive State*, London: Pinter.

Hirst, J. (1998) 'Yes, Minister – or else!' *Community Care*, 24–30 September: 8–9.

Hobsbawm, E. (1996) 'Identity politics and the left', *New Left Review* 217: 38–48.

Hodgkinson, P. (2000) 'Who wants to be a social engineer? A commentary on David Blunkett's speech to the ESRC', *Sociological Research Online* 5 (1), http://www.soresonline.org.uk/5/1/hodgkinson.html.

Hoghugi, M. and Speight, A. N. P. (1998) 'Good enough parenting for all children: a strategy for a healthier society', *Archives of Disease in Childhood* 78 (4): 293–300.

Holdaway, S. (1986) 'Police and social work relations: problems and possibilities', *British Journal of Social Work* 16: 137–60.

Holden, C. (2002) 'British government policy and the concentration of ownership in long-term care provision', *Ageing and Society* 22: 79–94.

Holman, B. (2000) 'Think local, Gordon', *Community Care*, 22–28 June: 22.

Home Office (1998) *Youth Justice: Preventing offending by Children and Young People*, London: HMSO.

Home Office (2000) 'New Guide to Crack Down on Anti-social Behaviour', press release, 29 June.

Home Office (2001) 'New steps towards an era of active citizenship', press release, 3 May.

Home Office (2002a) 'Thirty-day countdown to publish race equality schemes', press release, 11 May.

Home Office (2002b) *Entitlement Cards and Identity Fraud: a Consultation Paper*, London: Stationery Office.

Home Office, Crown Prosecution Service, Department of Health, Action for Justice (2001) *Provision of Therapy for Child Witnesses prior to a Criminal Trial: Practice Guide*, London: HMSO.

Home Office, Department of Health (2002) *Complex Child Abuse Investigations: Inter-agency Issues*, London: Home Office Communication Directorate.

Hopton, J. (1997) 'Anti-discriminatory practice and anti-oppressive practice', *Critical Social Policy* 17 (3): 47–61.

Hopton, J. (1999) 'Militarism, masculinism and managerialisation in the British public sector', *Journal of Gender* 8 (1): 71–82.

Hosegood, C. (1993) 'Issues in the adoption of Irish children', *Adoption and Fostering* 17 (1): 37–40.

Houston, S. (2002) 'Reflecting on habitus, field and capital: towards a culturally sensitive social work', *Journal of Social Work* 2 (2): 149–67.

Howard League for Penal Reform (2002a) 'Howard League granted permission in Children Act case', press release, 30 May.

Howard League for Penal Reform (2002b) 'Government reported to UN for breaching rights of children in prison', press release, 19 September.

Howard League for Penal Reform (2002c) 'Children in prison given protection under landmark ruling', press release, 29 November.

Howarth, J. (2000) 'Assessing the world of the child in need: background and context' in Department of Health, *The Child's World: Assessing Children in Need – Reader*, London: Department of Health.

Howarth, J. (ed.) (2001) *The Child's World: Assessing Children in Need*, London: Jessica Kingsley.

Howe, D. (1994) 'Modernity, postmodernity and social work', *British Journal of Social Work* 24: 513–32.

Howe, D., Sawbridge, P. and Hinings, D. (1992) *Half a Million Women: Mothers who lose their Children by Adoption*, Harmondsworth: Penguin.

Hughes, B. and Logan, J. (1995) 'The agenda for post-adoption services', *Fostering and Adoption* 19 (1): 34–7.

Hughes, B., Parker, H. and Gallagher, B. (1996) *Policing Child Sexual Abuse: the View of Police Practitioners*, London: Home Office.

Hughes, J. and Sharrock, W. (1997) *The Philosophy of Social Research*, London: Longman.

Humphreys, C. (1996) 'Exploring new territory: police organizational responses to child sexual abuse', *Child Abuse Review* 20: 332–44.

Humphries, B. (1997) 'Reading social work: competing discourses in the rules and requirements for the Diploma in Social Work', *British Journal of Social Work* 27: 641–58.

Hunter, M. (1999) 'Team spirit', *Community Care*, 17–23 June: 20–2.

Hunter, M. (2002) 'Star teams drop in', *Community Care*, 12–18 September: 32–4.

Hutton, J., Minister of State for Social Services (2000) Foreword in Department of Health, *Assessing Children in Need and their Families: Practice Guidance*, London: Stationery Office.

Hutton, J., Clarke, C. and Smith, J. (2000) *Framework for the Assessment of Children in Need and their Families*, circular from Department of Health, Home Office and Department for Education and Employment, 4 April.

Iarskaia-Smirnova, E. and Romanov, P. (2002) 'A salary is not important here: the professionalization of social work in contemporary Russia', *Social Policy and Administration* 36 (2): 123–41.

International Federation of Social Workers (2000) *Definition of Social Work* http://www.ifsw.org/Publications/4.6e.pub.html.

Irving, A. and Young, T. (2002) 'Paradigm for pluralism: Mikhail Bakhtin and social work practice', *Social Work* 47 (1): 19–30.

Jack, G. (2000a) 'Ecological influences on parenting and child development', *British Journal of Social Work* 30: 703–20.

Jack, G. (2000b) 'Ecological perspectives in assessing children and families' in Department of Health, *The Child's World: Assessing Children in Need – Reader*, London: Department of Health.

Jack, G. and Jordan, B. (1999) 'Social capital and child welfare', *Children and Society* 13: 242–56.

Jackson, P. (1998) 'Constructions of "whiteness" in the geographical imagination', *Area* 30 (2): 99–106.

Jackson, S. (1988–9) 'Residential care and education', *Children and Society* 4: 335–50.

Jackson, S. (1998) 'Looking after Children: a new approach or just an exercise in form filling? A response to Knight and Caveney', *British Journal of Social Work* 28: 45–56.

Jackson, S. and Kilroe, S. (eds) (1996) *Looking after Children: Good Parenting, Good Outcomes Reader*, London: HMSO.

Jackson, S., Fisher, M. and Ward, H. (1996) 'Key concepts in Looking after Children: parenting, partnership, outcomes' in S. Jackson and S. Kilroe (eds) *Looking after Children: Good Parenting, Good Outcomes Reader*, London: HMSO.

Jacques, M. (1998) 'Good to be back', *Marxism Today*, November–December: 2–3.

James, A. L. and James, A. (2001) 'Tightening the net: children, community and control', *British Journal of Sociology* 52 (2): 211–28.

James, A. and Jencks, C. (1996) 'Public perceptions of childhood criminality', *British Journal of Sociology* 47 (2): 315–32.

James, A. and Prout, A. (eds) (1996a) *Constructing and Reconstructing Childhood*, London: Falmer.

James, A. and Prout, A. (1996b) 'Re-presenting childhood: time and transition in the study of childhood' in A. James and A. Prout (eds) *Constructing and Reconstructing Childhood*, London: Falmer.

James, A., Jencks, C. and Prout, A. (1998) *Theorising Childhood*, Cambridge: Polity Press.

Jameson, F. (2000) 'Globalization and political strategy', *New Left Review* 4: 49–69.

Jerrom, C. (2001) 'Is a £2 m campaign enough to revitalise the social care work force?', *Community Care*, 18–24 October: 18–20.

Jerrom, C. (2002a) 'Will children be labelled "criminals" if panels are given green light?' *Community Care*, 31 October–6 November: 20–2.

Jerrom, C. (2002b) 'Number of young women in secure units rises by nearly half in a year', *Community Care*, 18–24 July: 14.

Johnson, T. (1993) 'Expertise and the state' in M. Gane and T. Johnson (eds) *Foucault's New Domains*, London: Routledge.

Jones, C. (1983) *State Social Work and the Working Class*, London: Macmillan.

Jones, C. (1996a) 'Regulating social work: a review of the review', in S. Jackson and M. Preston-Shoot (eds) *Educating Social Workers in a Changing Policy Context*, London: Whiting & Birch.

Jones, C. (1996b) 'Anti-intellectualism and the peculiarities of British social work education' in N. Parton (ed.) *Social Theory, Social Change and Social Work*, London: Routledge.

Jones, C. (2001) 'Voices from the Front Line: State Social Workers and New Labour', *British Journal of Social Work* 31: 547–62.

Jones, D. (2000) 'The assessment of parental capacity' in Department of Health, *The Child's World: Assessing Children in Need – Reader*, London: Department of Health.

Jones, D. A. (1999) 'Regulating social work: key questions', *Practice* 11 (3): 55–64.

Jones, H. (1997) (ed.) *Towards a Classless Society?* London: Routledge.

Jones, H., Clark, R., Kefeldt, K. and Norman, M. (1998) 'Looking after Children: assessing outcomes in child care: the experience of implementation', *Children and Society* 12: 212–22.

Jordan, B. (1974) *Poor Parents*, London: Routledge.

Jordan, B. (1998) *The New Politics of Welfare*, London: Sage.

Jordan, B. (2001) 'Tough love: social work, social exclusion and the Third Way', *British Journal of Social Work* 31: 527–46.

Jordan, B, with Jordan, C. (2000) *Social Work and the Third Way*, London: Sage.

Kamerman, S. B. and Kahn, A. J. (1990) 'If CPS is driving child welfare – where do we go from here?' *Public Welfare*, winter: 9–14.

Kanya-Forstner, M. (1999) 'Defining womanhood: Irish women and the Catholic Church in Victorian Liverpool', *Immigrants and Minorities* 18 (2–3): 168–89.

Katz, N. S. (2000) 'Dual systems of adoption in the United States' in S. N. Katz, J. Eekelaar and M. Maclean (eds) *Cross Currents: Family Law and Policy in the US and England*, Oxford: Oxford University Press.

Kay, J. (1991) *The Adoption Papers*, Newcastle upon Tyne: Bloodaxe.

Kelly, G. and Coulter, J. (1997) 'The Children (Northern Ireland) Order 1995: a new era for fostering and adoption services', *Adoption and Fostering* 21 (3): 5–14.

Kelly, S. and Blythe, B. J. (2000) 'Family preservation: a potential not yet realized', *Child Welfare*, January–February: 29–43.

Kemp, S. and Squires, J. (1997) *Feminisms*, Oxford: Oxford University Press.

Kendall, L. and Harker, L. (2002) *From Welfare to Wellbeing: the Future of Social Care*, London: IPPR.

Khan, P. and Dominelli, L. (2000) 'The impact of globalization on social work in the UK', *European Journal of Social Work* 3 (2): 95–108.

Kilroe, S. (1996) 'Social presentation' in S. Jackson and S. Kilroe (eds) *Looking after Children: Good Parenting, Good Outcomes Reader*, London: HMSO.

King, D. and Wickham-Jones, M. (1999) 'From Clinton to Blair: the Democratic (Party) origins of Welfare to Work', *Political Quarterly* 70 (1): 62–75.

Kirkby, P., Gibbons, L. and Cronin, M. (2002) 'The reinvention of Ireland: a critical perspective' in P. Kirkby, L. Gibbons and M. Cronin (eds) *Reinventing Ireland: Culture, Society and the Global Economy*, London: Pluto Press.

Kirkpatrick, I., Kitchener, M. and Whipp, R. (2001) 'Out of sight, out of mind: assessing the impact of markets for children's residential care', *Public Administration* 73 (1): 49–71.

Kirton, D. (1996) 'Race and adoption', *Critical Social Policy* 16 (1): 123–37.

Kirton, D. (1999) 'Perspectives in "race" and adoption: the views of student social workers', *British Journal of Social Work* 29: 779–96.

Kirton, D. (2000) *'Race', Ethnicity and Adoption*, Buckingham: Open University Press.

Klein, M. (2000) *No Logo*, London: Flamingo.

Knight, T. and Caveney, S. (1998) 'Assessment and Action Records: will they promote good parenting?' *British Journal of Social Work* 28: 29–43.

Krane, J. and Davies, L. (2000) 'Mothering and child protection practice: rethinking risk assessment', *Child and Family Social Work* 5: 35–45.

Kuhn, T. (1966) *The Structure of Scientific Revolutions*, Chicago: University of Chicago Press.

Kundnani, A. (2001) 'In a foreign land: the new popular racism', *Race and Class* 43 (2): 41–60.

Kvale, S. (1996) *InterViews*, London: Sage.

Ladipo, D. (2001) 'The rise of America's prison-industrial complex', *New Left Review* 7: 109–24.

Lang, T. (1997) 'Dividing up the cake: food as social exclusion' in A. Walker and C. Walker (eds) *Divided Britain: the Growth of Social Exclusion in Britain, 1979–1997*, London: Child Poverty Action Group.

Lardner, R. (1992) 'Factors affecting police/social work inter-agency co-operation in a Child Protection Unit', *Police Journal*, July: 213–29.

Lash, S. and Urry, J. (1999) *Economies of Sign and Space*, London: Sage.

Lea, J. (2000) 'The Macpherson report and the question of institutional racism', *Howard Journal* 39 (3): 219–33.

Leason, K. (2002) 'Unison local government conference backs motion opposing care trusts', *Community Care*, 20–26 June: 8.

Lee, N. (2001) *Childhood and Society*, Buckingham: Open University Press.

Leigh, M. (1997) *Secrets and Lies*, London: Faber.

Lentin, R. (2001) 'Responding to the racialisation of Irishness: disavowed multiculturalism and its discontents', *Sociological Research Online* 5 (4), http://www.socresonline.org.uk/5/4lentin.html.

Leonard, P. (2000) *Postmodern Welfare: Reconstructing an Emancipatory Project*, London: Sage.

Levitas, R. (1996) 'The concept of social exclusion and the new Durheimian hegemony', *Critical Social Policy* 16 (1): 5–21.

Lewis, G. (2000) 'Discursive histories, the pursuit of multiculturalism and social policy' in G. Lewis, S. Gerwitz and J. Clarke (eds) *Rethinking Social Policy*, London: Sage/Open University.

Lewis, J. (1986) 'Anxieties about the family and the relationships between parents, children and the state in twentieth-century England' in M. Richards and P. Light (eds) *Children of Social Worlds: Development in a Social Context*, Cambridge: Polity Press.

Lewis, A. and Lindsay, G. (eds) (2000) *Researching Children's Perspectives*, Buckingham: Open University Press.

Lindsay, M. (1998) 'Discrimination against young people in care: the theory of careism', *ChildRight*, November: 11–14.

Lister, R. (1997) *Citizenship: Feminist Perspectives*, Basingstoke: Macmillan.

Little, M. (1998) 'Whispers in the library: a response to Liz Trinder's article on the state of social work research', *Child and Family Social Work* 3: 49–56.

Lloyd, S. and Burman, M. (1996) 'Specialist police units and the joint investigation of child abuse', *Child Abuse Review* 5: 4–17.

Local Government Association, NHS Confederation, Association of Directors of Social Services (2002) *Serving Children Well: a New Vision for Children's Services*, London: LGA Publications.

Logan, J. (1996) 'Birth mothers and their mental health', *British Journal of Social Work* 26: 609–35.

Logan, J. and Hughes, B. (1995) 'The agenda for post-adoption services', *Adoption and Fostering* 19 (1): 34–7.

London, L. (2000) 'Whitehall and the refugees: the 1930s and the 1990s', *Patterns of Prejudice* 34 (3): 17–27.

London Borough of Bexley and Bexley Area Health Authority (1982) *Linda Gates and her Family*, London: London Borough of Bexley and Bexley Area Health Authority.

London Borough of Brent (1985) *A Child in Trust: the Report of the Panel of Inquiry into the Circumstances surrounding the Death of Jasmine Beckford*, London: London Borough of Brent.

London Borough of Greenwich (1987) *A Child in Mind: Protection of Children in a Responsible Society: the Report of the Commission of Inquiry into the Circumstances surrounding the Death of Kimberley Carlile*, London: London Borough of Greenwich.

London Borough of Lambeth (1987) *Whose Child? The Report of the Public Inquiry into the death of Tyra Henry*, London: London Borough of Lambeth.

Loos, R. (1994) 'No-go Britain', *Daily Mirror*, 20 April.

Lorenz, W. (1994) *Social Work in a Changing Europe*, London: Routledge.

Lorenz, W. (2000) 'Contentious identities: social work research and the search for professional and personal identities', *Theorising Social Research* seminar, 6 March, http://www.nisw.org.uk/tswr/lorenz.html.

Lowe, N. V. (2000) 'English adoption law: past, present and future' in S. N. Katz, J. Eekelaar and M. Maclean (eds) *Cross Currents: Family Law and Policy in the US and England*, Oxford: Oxford University Press.

Luster, T. and Okagaki, L. (1993) *Parenting: an Ecological Perspective*, Hillsdale NJ: Erlbaum.

Lyon, C. M. (1997) 'Children abused within the care system' in N. Parton (ed.) *Child Protection and Family Support*, London: Routledge.

Lyon, D. (2001a) *Surveillance Society: Monitoring Everyday Life*, Buckingham: Open University Press.

Lyon, D. (2001b) 'Surveillance after September 11', *Sociological Research Online* 6 (3), http://www.socresonline.org.uk/6/3/lyon.html.

Macdonald, G. (1999) 'Evidenced-based social care: wheels off the runway?' *Public Money and Management* 19 (1): 25–33.

Macdonald, G. and Roberts, H. (1995) *What Works in the Early Years?* Ilford: Barnardo's.

MacNicol, J. (1987) 'In pursuit of the underclass', *Journal of Social Policy* 16 (3): 293–318.

Macpherson, Sir William of Cluny (1999) *The Stephen Lawrence Inquiry*, London: Stationery Office.

Maddox, B. (1996) 'A fine old Irish stew', *New Statesman*, 29 November: 21–3.

Maguire, M. (1997) 'Missing links: working class women of Irish descent' in P. Mahony and C. Zmroczek (eds) *Class Matters: 'Working Class' Women's Perspectives on Social Class*, London: Taylor & Francis.

Malin, N. (ed.) (2000) *Professionalism, Boundaries and the Workplace*, London: Routledge.

Maluccio, A. N., Fein, E. and Olmstead, K. A. (1986) *Permanency Planning for Children: Concepts and Methods*, London: Tavistock.

Mann, K. (1994) 'Watching the defectives: observers of the underclass in the USA, Britain and Australia', *Critical Social Policy* 41: 79–100.

Mann, M. (2001) 'Globalisation after September 11', *New Left Review* 12: 51–73.

Marchant, R. (2000) 'The assessment of children with complex needs' in Department of Health, *The Child's World: Assessing Children in Need – Reader*, London: Department of Health.

Marchant, R. and Jones, M. (2000) 'Assessing the needs of disabled children and their families' in Department of Health, *Assessing Children in Need and their Families: Practice Guidance*, London: Stationery Office.

Margolin, L. (1997) *Under the Cover of Kindness: the Invention of Social Work*, Charlottesville, VA: University of Virginia Press.

Marston, S. A. (2002) 'Making a difference: conflict over Irish identity in the New York City St Patrick's Day parade', *Political Geography* 21: 373–92.

Martinez-Brawley, E. M. and Mendez-Bonito Zorito, P. (1998) 'At the edge of the frame: beyond science and art in social work', *British Journal of Social Work* 28: 197–212.

Mason, K. and Selman, P. (1997) 'Birth parents' experiences of contested adoption', *Adoption and Fostering* 21 (1): 21–9.

Mauther, M. (1997) 'Methodological aspects of collecting data from children: lessons from three research projects', *Children and Society* 11: 16–28.

May, T. (1993) *Social Research*, Buckingham: Open University Press.

May, T. and Buck, M. (1998) 'Power, professionalism and organisational transformation', *Sociological Research Online* 3 (1), http://www.socresonline.org.uk/3/2/5.html.

Maynard, M. (1994) 'Race, gender and the concept of difference in feminist thought' in H. Afshar and M. Maynard (eds) *The Dynamics of 'Race' and Gender*, London: Taylor & Francis.

Maza, P. L. (2000) 'Using administrative data to reward agency performance: the case of the Federal Adoption Incentive Programme', *Child Welfare* 79 (5): 444–57.

McBeath, G. B. and Webb, S. A. (1991) 'Social work, modernity and post-modernity', *Sociological Review* 39: 745–63.

McCurry, P. (1999a) 'In on the Act', *Community Care*, 1–7 April: 20–2.

McCurry, P. (1999b) 'Raring to go', *Community Care*, 21–7 October: 20–3.

McDonald, P. and Coleman, M. (1999) 'Deconstructing hierarchies of oppression and adopting a "multiple model" approach to anti-oppressive practice', *Social Work Education* 18 (1): 19–34.

McGowan, B. G. and Walsh, E. M. (2000) 'Policy challenges for child welfare in the new century', *Child Welfare*, January–February: 11–28.

McGregor, S. (1999) 'Welfare, neo-liberalism and the new paternalism: three ways for social policy in late capitalist societies', *Capital and Class* 67: 91–119.

McRoy, R. G. (1991) 'American experience and research on openness', *Adoption and Fostering* 15 (4): 99–111.

Mead, L. M. (ed.) (1997) *The New Paternalism: Supervisory Approaches to Poverty*, Washington DC: Brookings Institution.

Meiksins Wood, E. (1995) 'A chronology of the New Left and its successors, or: who's old-fashioned now?' in L. Panitch (ed.) *Socialist Register 1995*, London: Merlin Press.

Melkie, J. (1997) 'Estates from hell behind '90s riots', *Guardian*, 25 June.

Merrick, D. (1996) *Social Work and Child Abuse*, London: Routledge.

Milburn, A. (2002) 'Social services to be "better structured in the interests of the user" ', http://www.doh.gov.uk/speeches/ann-soc-serv-con-2002.htm.

Miles, R. (1993) *Racism after 'Race Relations'*, London: Routledge.

Miller, A. (1998) 'Bringing up Baby', *Community Care*, 13–19 August: 21.

Milner, J. (1993) 'A disappearing act: the differing career paths of fathers and mothers in child protection investigations', *Critical Social Policy* 13 (2): 48–64.

Milotte, M. (1997) *Banished Babies*, Dublin: New Island Books.

Ministerial Group on the Family (1998) *Supporting Families: a Consultative Document*, London: Stationery Office.

Mitchell, D. (1997) 'Minister lashes out against social work', *Community Care*, 3–9 July: 4.

Modood, T., Berthoud, R., Lakey, J., Nazroo, J., Smith, P., Virdee, S. and Beishon, S. (1997) *Ethnic Minorities in Britain: Diversity and Difference*, London: Policy Studies Institute.

Mooney, J. and Young, J. (1999) *Social Exclusion and Criminal Justice*, London: Centre for Criminology, Middlesex University.

Moore, J. (2002) 'Truants learned a lesson when mum went to jail', *Sun*, 29 May.

Moran Ellis, J., Conroy, S., Fielding, N. and Tunstill, J. (1991) *Investigation of Child Abuse: an Executive Summary*, London: Police Foundation.

Morgan, P. (1998) *Adoption and the Care of Children*. London: IEA Health and Welfare Unit.

Morgan, P. (1999) *Farewell to the Family: Public Policy and Family Breakdown in Britain and the USA*, 2nd edn, London: IEA Health and Welfare Unit.

Morrow, V. (1999) 'Conceptualising social capital in relation to the well-being of children and young people: a critical review', *Sociological Review* 47 (4): 744–66.

Moss, P., Dillon, J. and Statham, J. (2000) 'The "child in need" and the "rich child": discourses, constructions and practice', *Critical Social Policy* 20 (2): 233–54.

Mouffe, C. (2000) *The Democratic Paradox*, London: Verso.

Mounsey, J. (1975) 'Offences of criminal violence, cruelty and neglect against children in Lancashire' in A. W. Franklin (ed.), *Concerning Child Abuse*, Edinburgh: Churchill Livingstone.

Moyers, S. and Mason, A. (1995) 'Identifying standards of parenting' in H. Ward (ed.) *Looking after Children: Research into Practice*, London: HMSO.

Mullender, A. and Kearn, S. (1997) *'I'm here waiting': Birth Relatives' Views on Part 11 of the Adoption Contact Register for England and Wales*, London: BAAF.

Munro, E. (2001) 'Empowering looked-after children', *Child and Family Social Work* 6: 129–37.

Murray, C. (1990) *The Emerging British Underclass*, London: Institute of Economic Affairs.

Murray, C. (1994) 'The new Victorians . . . and the new rabble', *Sunday Times*, 29 May.

Navarro, V. (1999) 'Is there a Third Way? A response to Giddens's *The Third Way*', *International Journal of Health Services* 29 (4): 667–77.

Nellis, M. (1999) 'Towards the "Field of Corrections": modernizing the probation service in the late 1990s', *Social Policy and Administration* 33 (3): 302–23.

Neocleous, M. (1999) 'Radical conservatism, or the conservatism of radicals: Giddens, Blair and the politics of reaction', *Radical Philosophy* 93, January–February: 24–35.

Neustatter, A. (2002) 'Prison can be the right place for kids', *New Statesman*, 19 August: 12–14.

Newburn, T. (1996) 'Back to the future? Youth crime, youth justice and the rediscovery of authoritarian populism' in J. Pilcher and S. Wagg (ed.) *Thatcher's Children? Politics, Childhood and Society in the 1980s and 1990s*, London: Falmer.

Newburn, T. (2002) 'Atlantic crossings: "policy transfer" and crime control in the USA and Britain', *Punishment and Society* 4 (2): 165–94.

Newman, J. (2001) *Modernising Governance: New Labour, Policy and Society*, London: Sage.

Newman, W. A. (1951) 'Legal adoption', *Bell* 16 (4): 59–66.

Ngabonziza, D. (1988) 'Inter-country adoption: in whose best interests?' *Adoption and Fostering* 12 (1): 35–41.

Ngabonziza, D. (1991) 'Moral and political issues facing relinquishing countries', *Adoption and Fostering* 15 (4): 75–81.

Nixon, J., Walker, M. and Baron, S. (2002) 'From Washington Heights to the Raploch: evidence, mediation, and the genealogy of policy', *Social Policy and Society* 1 (3): 237–47.

Norman, A. (1985) *Triple Jeopardy: Growing Old in a Second Homeland*, London: Centre for Policy on Ageing.

Nuccio, K. E. and Sands, R. G. (1992) 'Using postmodern feminist theory to deconstruct "phallacies" of poverty', *Affilia* 7 (4): 26–48.

O'Brian, C. (1997/8) 'International adoption from China', *Adoption and Fostering* 21 (4): 6–14.

O'Brien, M., Penna, S. and Hay, C. (eds) (1999) *Theorising Modernity*, Harlow: Addison Wesley Longman.

Oldman, D. (1994) 'Adult–child relations as class relations' in J. Qvortrup (ed.) *Childhood Matters*, Aldershot: Avebury.

Oliver, M. (1984) 'The politics of disability', *Critical Social Policy* 11: 21–33.

O'Neale, V. (2000) *Excellence not Excuses: Inspection of Services for Ethnic Minority Children and Families*, London: Department of Health.

Orkneys report (1992) *The Report of the Inquiry into the Removal of Children from Orkney in February 1991*, Edinburgh: HMSO.

Orme, J. (2001) 'Regulation or fragmentation? Directions for social work under New Labour', *British Journal of Social Work* 31: 611–24.

O'Sullivan, J. (1996) 'If you're hip, you must be Irish', *Independent*, 1 July.

Palme, C. (1999) 'Adopting an Irish identity', *Irish Post*, 10 October.

Pardeck, J. T., Murphy, J. W. and Min Choi, J. (1994) 'Some implications of post-modernism for social work practice', *Social Work* 39 (4): 343–7.

Parekh report (2000) *The Future of Multi-ethnic Britain*, London: Runnymede Trust.

Parker, H., Gallagher, B. and Hughes, B. (1996) 'The policing of child sexual abuse in England and Wales', *Policing and Society* 6: 1–13.

Parker, J. (2000) 'Social work with refugees and asylum seekers: a rationale for developing practice', *Practice* 12 (3): 61–77.

Parker, R., Ward, H., Jackson, S., Aldgate, J. and Wedge, P. (1991) *Looking after Children: Assessing Outcomes in Child Care*, London: HMSO.

Parton, N. (1985) *The Politics of Child Abuse*, London: Macmillan.

Parton, N. (1990) 'Taking child abuse seriously' in Violence against Children Study Group, *Taking Child Abuse Seriously*, London: Unwin Hyman.

Parton, N. (1991) *Governing the Family: Child Care, Child Protection and the State*, London: Macmillan.

Parton, N. (1994) 'Problematics of government, (post)modernity and social work', *British Journal of Social Work* 24: 9–32.

Parton, N. (1995) 'Neglect as child protection: the political context and the practical outcomes', *Children and Society* 9 (1): 67–89.

Parton, N. (1998) 'Risk, advanced liberalism and child welfare: the need to rediscover uncertainty and ambiguity', *British Journal of Social Work* 28: 5–28.

Parton, N. (1999) 'Some thoughts on the relationship between theory and practice in and for social work', *Theorising Social Work Research* seminar, 26 May, http://www.nisw.org.uk/tswr/parton.html.

Parton, N. and Marshall, W. (1998) 'Postmodernism and discourse approaches to social work' in R. Adams, L. Dominelli and M. Payne (eds) *Social Work: Themes, Issues and Critical Debates*, London: Macmillan.

Parton, N. and O'Byrne, P. (2000) *Constructive Social Work*, London: Macmillan.

Payne, M. (1997) *Modern Social Work Theory*, 2nd edn, London: Macmillan.

Payne, M. (2000) *Teamwork in Multiprofessional Care*, London: Macmillan.

Pearce, J. (2001a) 'Holes in the safety net', *Community Care*, 22–28 March: 12.

Pearce, J. (2001b) 'Social fund undermining bid to end child poverty', *Community Care*, 12–18 April: 8–9.

Pearce, J. (2001c) 'Government refutes need to overhaul Social Fund', *Community Care*, 16–22 August: 6–7.

Pearson, M., Madden, M. and Greenslade, L. (1991) *Generations of Invisibility: the Health and Well-being of the Irish in Britain*, Liverpool: Institute of Irish Studies, University of Liverpool.

Pease, B. and Fook, J. (1999) 'Postmodern critical theory and emancipatory social work practice' in B. Pease and J. Fook (eds) *Transforming Social Work Practice: Postmodern Critical Perspectives*, London: Routledge.

Peck, J. (1998) 'Workfare: a geopolitical etymology', *Environment and Planning D: Society and Space* 16: 133–61.

Peile, C. and McCourt, M. (1997) 'The rise of relativism: the future of theory and knowledge development in social work', *British Journal of Social Work*, 27: 343–60.

Performance and Innovation Unit (2000) *The Prime Minister's Review of Adoption: a Performance and Innovation Unit Report*, London: Stationery Office.

Philp, A. F. and Timms, N. (1957) *The Problem of the 'Problem Family'*, London: Family Service Unit.

Philpot, T. (2002) 'Duncan Smith puts the case for less state and more common sense', *Community Care*, 3–9 October: 20–2.

Phoenix, A. (1998) 'Dealing with difference: the recursive and the new', *Ethnic and Racial Studies* 21 (5): 859–81.

Pierson, C. and Castles, F. G. (2002) 'Australian antecedents of the Third Way', *Political Studies* 50: 683–702.

Pilkington, A. (2003) *Racial Disadvantage and Ethnic Diversity in Britain*, London: Palgrave Macmillan.

Pinnock, M. and Garnett, L. (2002) 'Needs-led or needs must?' in H. Ward and W. Rose (eds) *Approaches to Needs Assessment in Children's Services*, London: Jessica Kingsley.

Pithouse, A. (1998) *Social Work: the Social Organisation of an Invisible Trade*, Aldershot: Ashgate.

Platt, D. (2002) 'Why stars are underrated', *Community Care*, 27 June–3 July: 36–9.

Polansky, N. A., Ammons, P. W. and Weathersby, B. L. (1983) 'Is there an American standard of child care?' *Social Work* 23 (5): 341–7.

Pollitt, C. (1993) *Managerialism and the Public Services*, Oxford: Blackwell.

Pooley, C. G. (1999) 'From Londonderry to London: identity and sense of place for Protestant Northern Irish women in the 1930s', *Immigrants and Minorities*, 18 (2–3): 189–214.

Poster, M. (1990) *The Mode of Information: Post-structuralism and Social Context*, Cambridge: Polity Press.

Powell, F. (2001) *The Politics of Social Work*, London: Sage.

Powell, M. (ed.) (1999) *New Labour, New Welfare State?* Bristol: Policy Press.

Powell, M. (2000) 'New Labour and the Third Way in the British welfare state: a new and distinctive approach?' *Critical Social Policy* 20 (1): 39–61.

Pozatek, E. (1994) 'The problem of certainty: clinical social work in the post-modern era', *Social Work* 39 (4): 396–404.

Prasad, R. (2001) 'Life support system', *Guardian Society*, 4 April.

Prideaux, S. (2001) 'New Labour, old functionalism: the underlying contradictions of Welfare reform in the US and the UK', *Social Policy and Administration* 35 (1): 85–115.

Prince, M. J. (2001) 'How social is social policy? Fiscal and market discourse in North American Welfare systems', *Social Policy and Administration* 35 (1): 2–13.

Pritchard, C. (1998) 'Matters of life and death', *Community Care*, 14–20 May: 20–1.

Prout, A. (2000) 'Children's participation: control and self-realisation in British late modernity', *Children and Society* 14: 304–15.

Prout, A. and James, A. (1990) 'A new paradigm for the sociology of childhood? Provenance, promise and problems' in A. James and A. Prout (eds) *Constructing and Reconstructing Childhood*, London: Falmer.

Pugh, R. and Gould, N. (2000) 'Globalization, social work and social welfare', *European Journal of Social Work* 3 (2): 123–38.

Quinton, D. (1996) 'Outcome measurement in work with children: a response to Huxley', *Child Abuse Review* 5: 83–9.

Quinton, D. and Murray, C. (2002) 'Assessing the emotional and behavioural development in children looked after away from home' in H. Ward and W. Rose (eds) *Approaches to Needs Assessment in Children's Services*, London: Jessica Kingsley.

Qvortrup, J. (1994) 'Childhood matters: an introduction' in J. Qvortrup (ed.) *Childhood Matters: Social Theory, Practice and Politics*, Aldershot: Avebury.

Reich, R. B. (2001) *The Future of Success: Work and Life in the New Economy*, London: Heinemann.

Reiner, R. (2000) *The Politics of the Police*, 3rd edn, Oxford: Oxford University Press.

Richmond, M. E. (1917) *Social Diagnosis*, New York: Russell Sage Foundation.

Rickford, F. (2000) 'Holding on to the past', *Community Care*, 1–7 June: 24–5.

Rickford, F. (2001) 'The bringing up baby blues', *Community Care*, 14–20 June: 20–2.

Rickford, F. (2002a) 'Eastern promise', *Community Care*, 28 March–3 April: 28–32.

Rickford, F. (2002b) 'Laming hears hindsight view of Haringey social services department', *Community Care*, 25–31 July: 18–20.

Rickford, F. (2002c) 'Denham signals move to use crime as the hook for children's policies', *Community Care*, 21–7 November: 20–2.

Roberts, H. and Welland, S. (1997) 'Hear my voice', *Community Care*, 16–22 January: 24–6.

Robinson, F. and Gregson, N. (1992) 'The "underclass": a class apart?' *Critical Social Policy* 34: 38–52.

Robinson, G. (2001) 'Power, knowledge and "what works" in probation', *Howard Journal* 40 (3): 235–54.

Rodger, J. J. (1991) 'Discourse analysis and social relationships in social work', *British Journal of Social Work* 21: 63–79.

Rodger, J. (1992) 'The welfare state and social closure: social division and the "underclass"', *Critical Social Policy* 35: 45–64.

Rogers, A. and Pilgrim, D. (1989) 'Mental health and citizenship', *Critical Social Policy* 26: 44–56.

Rogers, C. (1980) *A Way of Being*, Boston, MA: Houghton Mifflin.

Rojek, C. (1986) 'The "subject" in social work', *British Journal of Social Work* 16: 65–77.

Rojek, C. and Collins, S. (1987) 'Contract or con trick?' *British Journal of Social Work* 17: 199–211.

Rooff, M. (1972) *A Hundred Years of Family Welfare*, London: Michael Joseph.

Rose, N. (1985) *The Psychological Complex: Psychology, Politics and Society in England, 1869–1939*, London: Routledge.

Rose, N. (1989) *Governing the Soul: the Shaping of the Private Self*, London: Routledge.

Rose, N. (1993) 'Government, authority and expertise in advanced liberalism', *Economy and Society* 22 (3): 283–300.

Rose, N. (1996) 'Governing "advanced" liberal democracies', in A. Barry, T. Osborne and N. Rose (eds) *Foucault and Political Reason*, London: UCL Press.

Rose, N. (1998) *Inventing Ourselves*, Cambridge: Cambridge University Press.

Rose, N. (1999) 'Inventiveness in politics', *Economy and Society* 28 (3): 467 94.

Rose, N. (2000) 'The biology of culpability', *Theoretical Criminology* 4 (1): 5–34.

Rose, N. and Miller, P. (1992) 'Political power beyond the state: problematics of government', *British Journal of Sociology* 43: 173–206.

Rose, W. (2000) 'Assessing children in need and their families: an overview of the framework' in Department of Health, *The Child's World: Assessing Children in Need – Reader*, London: Department of Health.

Rose, W. (2002) 'Two steps forward, one step back' in H. Ward and W. Rose (eds) *Approaches to Needs Assessment in Children's Services*, London: Jessica Kingsley.

Rose, W. and Aldgate, J. (2000) 'Knowledge underpinning the Assessment Framework' in Department of Health, *Assessing Children in Need and their Families: Practice Guidance*, London: Stationery Office.

Rosenau, P. M. (1992) *Postmodernism and the Social Sciences*, Chichester: Princeton University Press.

Roskill, C. (2000) 'Lest we forget', *Community Care*, 26 October: 26–8.

Rossiter, A. (2000) 'The postmodern feminist condition: new conditions for social work', in B. Fawcett, B. Featherstone, J. Fook and A. Rossiter (eds) *Practice and Research in Social Work: Postmodern Feminist Perspectives*, London: Routledge.

Roth, J. (1980) *The Lost Children: a Study of Charity Children in Ireland, 1700–1900*, Dublin: Institute of Public Administration.

Rustin, M. (1994) 'Incomplete modernity: Ulrich Beck's risk society', *Radical Philosophy* 67: 3–13.

Ryburn, M. (1992) 'Contested adoption proceedings', *Adoption and Fostering* 16 (4): 29–39.

Ryburn, M. (1994) *Open Adoption: Research, Theory and Practice*. Aldershot: Avebury.

Sales, R. (2002) 'The deserving and undeserving? Refugees, asylum seekers and Welfare in Britain', *Critical Social Policy* 22 (3): 456–79.

Sanders, R, Jackson, S. and Thomas, T. (1996) 'The police role in the management of child protection services', *Policing and Society* 6. 87–100.

Sanderson, R. (2002) 'Evaluation, policy learning and evidence-based policy making', *Public Administration* 80 (1): 1–22.

Sandland, R. (1993) 'Adoption, law and homosexuality: can gay people adopt a child?' *Journal of Social Welfare and Family Law* 5: 321–33.

Schechter, M. D. and Bertocci, D. (1990) 'The meaning of the search' in D. M. Brodzinsky and M. D. Schechter (eds) *The Psychology of Adoption*, Oxford: Oxford University Press.

Scottish Executive (2002) *Scotland's Action Programme to Reduce Youth Crime 2002*, Edinburgh: Stationery Office.

Scourfield, J. (2000) 'The rediscovery of child neglect', *Sociological Review* 48 (3): 365–83.

Scraton, P. (ed.) (1987) *Law and the Authoritarian State*, Milton Keynes: Open University Press.

Scraton, P. (1997) (ed.) *Childhood in Crisis?* London: UCL Press.

Secretary of State for Health (1998a) *The Government's Response to the Children's Safeguards Review*, London: Stationery Office.

Secretary of State for Health (1998b) *Quality Protects: Transforming Children's Services: The Role and Responsibilities of Councillors*. London: Department of Health.

Secretary of State for Social Services (1988) *Report of the Inquiry into Child Abuse in Cleveland*, London: HMSO.

Segal, L. (1987) *Is the Future Female? Troubled Thoughts on Contemporary Feminism*, London: Virago.

Segal, L. (1990) *Slow Motion: Changing Masculinities Changing Men*, London: Virago.

Seita, J. R. (2000) 'In our best interests: three necessary shifts for child welfare workers and children', *Child Welfare*, January–February: 77–93.

Selwyn, J. (1996) 'Ascertaining children's wishes and feelings in relation to adoption', *Adoption and Fostering* 20 (3): 14–21.

Sennett, R. (1999) *The Corrosion of Character: the Personal Consequences of Work in the New Capitalism*, London: Norton.

Shamgar-Handelman, L. (1994) 'To whom does childhood belong?' in J. Qvortrup (ed.) *Childhood Matters: Social Theory, Practice and Politics*, Aldershot: Avebury.

Shaw, C. R. and McKay, H. D. (1969) *Juvenile Delinquency and Urban Areas*, 2nd edn, Chicago: University of Chicago Press.

Shaw, I. and Shaw, A. (1997) 'Keeping social work honest: evaluating as profession and practice', *British Journal of Social Work* 27: 847–69.

Shemmings, Y. and Shemmings, D. (2000) 'Empowering children and family members to participate in the assessment process' in Department of Health, *The Child's World: Assessing Children in Need – Reader*, London: Department of Health.

Sheppard, M. (1998) 'Practice validity, reflexivity and knowledge for social work', *British Journal of Social Work* 28: 763–81.

Shepherd, M. and Watkins, M. (2000) 'The Parent Concerns Questionnaire: evaluation of a mothers' self-report instrument for the identification of problems and needs in child and family social work', *Children and Society* 14: 194–206.

Siegel, D. H. (1993) 'Open adoption of infants: adoptive parents' perceptions of advantages and disadvantages', *Social Work* 38 (1): 15–24.

Simpkin, M. (1983) *Trapped within Welfare: Surviving Social Work*, London: Macmillan.

Sinclair, R. and Bullock, R. (2002) *Learning from Past Experience: A Review of Serious Case Reviews*, London: Department of Health.

Sinclair, R. and Little, M. (2002) 'Developing a taxonomy for children in need' in H. Ward and W. Rose (eds) *Approaches to Needs Assessment in Children's Services*, London: Jessica Kingsley.

Singh, G. (1997) 'Developing critical perspectives in Anti-racist and Anti-oppressive Theory and Practice – into the new millennium', paper delivered at the National Organisation of Practice Teachers' annual conference, University of Manchester Institute of Science and Technology, 9–11 July.

Sivanandan, A. (1998–9) 'Globalism and the left', *Race and Class* 44 (2–3): 5–20.

Sivanandan, A. (2000) 'Reclaiming the struggle', *Race and Class* 42 (2): 67–74.

Skeggs, B. (1997) *Formations of Class and Gender*, London: Sage.

Smale, G. and Tuson, G. with Biehal, N. and Marsh, P. (1993) *Empowerment, Assessment, Care Management and the Skilled Worker*, London: National Institute for Social Work/HMSO.

Small, J. (1982) 'New black families', *Adoption and Fostering* 6 (3): 35–40.

Small, J. with Prevatt Goldstein, B. (2000) 'Ethnicity and placement: beginning the debate', *Adoption and Fostering* 24 (1): 9–15.

Smart, C. (ed.) (1992) *Regulating Womanhood: Historical Essays on Marriage, Motherhood and Sexuality*, London: Routledge.

Smiley, M. (2001) 'Welfare dependence: the power of a concept', *Thesis Eleven* 64: 21–38.

Smith, C. (1997) 'Children's rights: have carers abandoned values?' *Children and Society* 11: 3–15.

Smith, C. (2000) 'The sovereign state *v.* Foucault: law and disciplinary power', *Sociological Review* 48 (2): 283–306.

Smith, C. and White, S. (1997) 'Parton, Howe and postmodernity: a critical comment on mistaken identity', *British Journal of Social Work* 27: 275–95.

Smith, D. J. and Gray, J. (1983) *Police and People in London* IV, *The Police in Action*, London: Policy Studies Institute.

Smith, G. (2000) 'Meeting the placement needs of Jewish children', *Adoption and Fostering* 24 (1): 40 7.

Smith, K. (2002) 'Scots staff to monitor children in bid to arrest delinquent behaviour', *Community Care*, 14–20 February: 16.

Smith, S. R. (1999) 'Arguing against cuts in lone parent benefits: reclaiming desert ground in the UK', *Critical Social Policy* 19 (3): 313–35.

Social Exclusion Unit (1999) *Bridging the Gap: New Opportunities for 16–18 year olds not in Education, Employment or Training*, London: Stationery Office.

Social Services Inspectorate (1997) *An Inspection of Local Authority Post-placement and Post-adoption Services*, London: HMSO.

Social Services Inspectorate (2000a) *LAC (98) 20: Adoption – Achieving the Right Balance: Response to Issues arising from SSI Survey of Local Authority Social Service Departments' Implementation of the Circular*, CI (2000) 7, London: Department of Health.

Social Services Inspectorate (2000b) *Adopting Changes: Survey and Inspection of local council's Adoption Services*, CI (2000) 22, London: Department of Health.

Social Services Inspectorate (2000c) *Modern Social Services: a Commitment to People: the Ninth Annual Report of the Chief Inspector of Social Services, 1999/2000*. London: Department of Health.

Social Services Inspectorate (2001) *Modern Social Services: a Commitment to Deliver*, London: Department of Health.

Social Services Inspectorate (2002) *A Guide to Social Services Performance 'Star' Ratings*, London: Department of Health.

Solinger, R. (2000) *Wake up, Little Susie: Single Pregnancy and Race before Roe v. Wade*, 2nd edn, London: Routledge.

Sone, K. (1996) 'A family law', *Community Care*, 31 October–6 November: 12.

Sone, K. (1997a) 'Moving stories', *Community Care*, 30 January–5 February: 20–1.

Sone, K. (1997b) 'No entry', *Community Care*, 25 September–1 October: 20–2.

Sparrow, P., Brooks, G. and Webb, D. (2002) 'National standards for the Probation Service: managing post-Fordist penality', *Howard Journal* 41 (1): 27–40.

Spinley, B. M. (1953) *The Deprived and the Privileged*, London: Routledge.

Spratt, T. and Houston, S. (1999) 'Developing critical social work in theory and in practice: child protection and communicative reason', *Child and Family Social Work* 4: 315–24.

Staffordshire County Council (1991) *The Pin-down Experience and the Protection of Children*, Stafford: Staffordshire County Council.

Starkey, P. (2000) 'The feckless mother: women, poverty and social workers in wartime and post-war England', *Women's History Review* 9 (3): 539–59.

Steele, L. (1998) 'Keeping a precarious balance', *Community Care*, 10–16 September: 2–9.

Stenson, K. (1993) 'Community policing as a governmental technology', *Economy and Society* 22 (3): 373–90.

Stevens, L., Brown, S. and Maclaren, P. (2000) 'Gender, nationality and cultural representations of Ireland', *European Journal of Women's Studies* 7: 405–21.

Stevenson, O. (1998) '"It was more difficult than we thought": a reflection on fifty years of child welfare practice', *Child and Family Social Work* 3: 153–61.

Stewart, G. and Stewart, J. (1986) *Boundary Changes: Social Work and Social Security*, London: Child Poverty Action Group.

Stone, S. (1994) 'Contact between adopters and birth parents: the Strathclyde experience', *Adoption and Fostering* 19 (2): 36–9.

Strangleman, T. (1999) 'The nostalgia of organisations and the organisation of nostalgia: past and present in the contemporary railway industry', *Sociology* 33 (4): 725–46.

Straw, J. and Anderson, J. (1996) *Parenting*, London: Labour Party.

Swanson, J. (2000) 'Self-help, Clinton, Blair and the politics of personal responsibility', *Radical Philosophy* 101, May–June: 29–39.

Taylor, A. (2001) 'Where the hurt is', *Community Care*, 14–20 June: 16.

Taylor, C. and White, S. (2000) *Practising Reflexivity in Health and Welfare*, Buckingham: Open University.

Taylor, C. and White, S. (2001) 'Knowledge, truth and reflexivity: the problem of judgement in social work', *Journal of Social Work* 1 (1): 37–59.

Taylor, I. (1999) *Crime in Context*, London: Cambridge.

Taylor, J., Spencer, N. and Baldwin, N. (2000) 'Social, economic and political context of parenting', *Archives of Disease in Childhood* 82 (2): 113–20.

Taylor-Gooby, P. (2000) 'Blair's scars', *Critical Social Policy* 20 (3): 331–449.

Taylor-Gooby, P. (2001) 'Risk, continuity and the Third Way: evidence from BHPS and qualitative studies', *Social Policy and Administration* 35 (2): 195–211.

Teague, A. (1989) *Social Change, Social Work and the Adoption of Children*, Aldershot: Avebury Gower.

Thoburn, J., Norford, L. and Parvez Rashid, S. (2000) *Permanent Family Placement for Children of Minority Ethnic Origin*, London: Jessica Kingsley.

Thomas, T. (1986) *The Police and Social Workers*, Aldershot: Gower.

Thomas, T. (1994) *The Police and Social Workers*, 2nd edn, Aldershot: Arena.

Thompson, A. (1998) 'The lost children', *Community Care*, 14–20 May: 18–19.

Thompson, N. (1997) *Anti-discriminatory Practice*, London: Macmillan.

Thompson, S. (2001) 'Introduction: towards an Irish cultural studies', *Cultural Studies* 15 (1): 1–11.

Tice, K. W. (1998) *Tales of Wayward Girls and Immoral Women: Case Records and the Professionalization of Social Work*, Urbana and Chicago: University of Illinois.

Tilki, M. (1998) 'The health of the Irish in Britain' in I. Papadopoulos, M. Tilki and G. Taylor (eds) *Transcultural Care: a Guide for Health Professionals*, Dinton: Quay Books.

Travers, T. (2001) 'Reach for the stars', *Public Finance* 16: 21–3.

Trinder, L. (2000) 'Reading the texts: postmodern feminism and the "doing" of research' in B. Fawcett, B. Featherstone, J. Fook and A. Rossiter (eds) *Practice and Research in Social Work: Postmodern Feminist Perspectives*, London: Routledge.

Triseliotis, J. (1973) *In Search of Origins: the Experience of Adopted People*, London: Routledge.

Triseliotis, J. (1991) 'Inter-country adoption', *Adoption and Fostering* 15 (4): 46–53.

Turney, D. (2000) 'The feminizing of neglect', *Child and Family Social Work* 5: 47–56.

Ullah, P. (1985) 'Second-generation Irish youth: identity and ethnicity', *New Community* 12: 35–50.

Unison (2002) 'Social services heading for meltdown, warns Unison', press notice, 28 May.

US Department of Health and Human Services, Administration for Children and Families (2000) 'HSS issues final child welfare regulations to improve services and outcomes for children', press notice, 25 January.

Utting, W. (1997) *People Like Us: Summary Report of the Review of the Safeguards for Children Living away from Home*, London: Department of Health/Welsh Office.

Valentine, G. (1996) 'Angels and devils: moral landscapes of childhood', *Environment and Planning D* 14: 581–99.

Valios, N. (1997) 'Report blasts politically correct adoption myths', *Community Care*, 16–22 October: 5.

Valios, N. (1998) 'Staff hit back at allegations of obsession with political dogma', *Community Care*, 23–29 April: 6–7.

Valios, N. (1999) 'Surfing a wave of controversy', *Community Care*, 28 October–3 November: 10–11.

Valios, N. (2000a) 'Charity calls for adopters' register', *Community Care*, 13–19 April: 2–3.

Valios, N. (2000b) 'Overhaul of legislation on cards', *Community Care*, 27 April–3 May: 2–3.

Valios, N. (2001) 'Burden of proof', *Community Care*, 8–14 March: 28–9.

Valios, N. (2002) 'UK in the dock', *Community Care*, 12–18 September: 28–30.

Van de Flier Davis, D. (1995) 'Capitalising on adoption', *Adoption and Fostering* 19 (2): 25–31.

Vaughan, B. (2000) 'The government of youth: disorder and dependence?' *Social and Legal Studies* 9 (3): 347–66.

Vaux, G. (2000) 'Hoorays and boos for Sure Start', *Community Care*, 30 March–5 April: 27.

Victor, P., Cooper, G. and Taylor, D. (1994) 'Fear rules in no-go Britain', *Independent on Sunday*, 17 April.

Virilio, P. (1997) *Open Sky*, London: Verso.

Wacquant, L. (2002) 'Slavery to mass incarceration', *New Left Review* 13: 41–61.

Waldfogel, J. (1998) *The Future of Child Protection*, Cambridge MA: Harvard University Press.

Waldfogel, J. (2000) 'Reforming child protective services', *Child Welfare*, January–February: 43–58.

Walker, C. and Walker, A. (1998) 'Social policy and social work' in R. Adams, L. Dominelli and M. Payne (eds) *Social Work, Themes, Issues and Critical Debates*, London: Macmillan.

Walker, R. (1999) 'The Americanization of British Welfare: a case study of policy transfer', *International Journal of Health Services* 29 (4): 679–97.

Walsh, C. (2002) 'Curfews: no more hanging around', *Youth Justice* 2 (2): 70–82.

Walshaw, R. S. (1941) *Migration to and from the British Isles*, London: Jonathan Cape.

Walter, B. (1995) 'Irishness, gender and place', *Society and Space* 13: 35–50.

Walter, B. (2000) 'Shamrocks growing out of their mouths: language and the racialisation of the Irish in Britain' in A. J. Kersten (ed.) *Language, Labour and Migration*, Aldershot: Ashgate.

Walter, B. (2001) *Outsiders Inside: Whiteness, Place and Irish Women*, London: Routledge.

Walter, B. with Gray, B., Almeida Dowling, L. and Morgan, S. (2002) *A Study of the existing Sources of Information and Analysis about Irish Emigrants and Irish Communities abroad*, Dublin: Government of Ireland Department of Foreign Affairs, www.gov.ie/iveagh.

Ward, H. (1993) 'Assessment and the Children Act 1989: the Looking after Children project' in H. Ferguson, R. Gilligan and R. Torode (eds) *Surviving Childhood Adversity: Issues for Policy and Practice*, Dublin: Social Studies Press/ Trinity College.

Ward, H. (ed.) (1995a) *Looking after Children: Research into Practice*, London: HMSO.

Ward, H. (1995b) 'Research and development strategy, 1991–1994' in H. Ward (ed.) *Looking after Children: Research into Practice*, London: HMSO.

Ward, H. (1995c) 'Revising the content of the Assessment and Action Records' in H. Ward (ed.) *Looking after Children: Research into Practice*, London: HMSO.

Ward, H. (1996) 'The Looking after Children package', *Child Care in Practice* 2 (4): 74–83.

Ward, H. (1998) 'Using a child development model to assess the outcomes of social work interventions with families', *Children and Society* 12: 202–11.

Ward, H. (2000a) 'Translating messages from research on child development into social work training and practice', *Social Work Education* 19 (6): 543–52.

Ward, H. (2000b) 'The development needs of children: implications for assessment' in Department of Health, *The Child's World: Assessing Children in Need – Reader*, London: Department of Health.

Ward, H. (2002) Introduction in H. Ward and W. Rose (eds) *Approaches to Needs Assessment in Children's Services*, London: Jessica Kingsley.

Ward, H. and Peel, M. (2002) 'An inter-agency approach to needs assessment' in H Ward and W. Rose (eds) *Approaches to Needs Assessment in Children's Services*, London: Jessica Kingsley.

Ward, H. and Skuse, T. (2001) 'Performance targets and the stability of placements for children long looked after away from home', *Children and Society* 15: 333–46.

Washington, J. and Paylor, I. (1998) 'Europe, social exclusion and the identity of social work', *British Journal of Social Work* 1 (3): 327–38.

Waterhouse, L. and Carnie, J. (1990a) 'Investigating child sexual abuse: towards inter-agency co-operation', *Adoption and Fostering* 14 (4): 7–13.

Waterhouse, L. and Carnie, J. (1990b) *Child Sexual Abuse: the Professional Challenge to Social Work and Police*, Edinburgh: University of Edinburgh.

Waterhouse, L. and Carnie, J. (1991) 'Research note: social work and police response to child sexual abuse in Scotland', *British Journal of Social Work* 21: 373–9.

Waterhouse, R. (2000) *Lost in Care: Report of the Tribunal of Inquiry into the Abuse of Children in Care in the former County Council Areas of Gwynedd and Clywd since 1974*, London: Stationery Office.

Watson, D. (2002) 'A critical perspective on quality with personal social services: prospects and concerns', *British Journal of Social Work* 32: 877 91.

Webb, D. (1996) 'Regulation for radicals: the state, CCETSW and the academy' in Parton, N. (ed.) *Social Theory, Social Change and Social Work*, London: Routledge.

Webb, R. and Vulliamy, G. (2001) 'Joining up the solutions: the rhetoric and practice of inter-agency co-ooperation', *Children and Society* 15: 315–32.

Webb, S. A. (2001) 'Some considerations on the validity of evidenced-based practice in social work', *British Journal of Social Work* 31: 57–79.

Webb, S. A. (2002) 'Local Orders and Global Chaos in Social Work', unpublished paper given at the thirtieth biannual conference of the International Association of Schools of Social Work (IASSW) 'Citizenship and Social Work Education in a Globalising World', University of Montpellier, 15 18 July.

Webb, S. A. and McBeath, G. B. (1989) 'A political critique of Kantian ethics in social work', *British Journal of Social Work* 19: 491–506.

Weinstock, A. (2000) Address to the Institute of Careers Guidance, http://www.uuy.org.uk/projects/connexio/weinstock_speech.htm.

Welland, S. (1999) 'Councils may lose grip on adoption services', *Community Care*, 1–7 April: 10.

Wells, S. (1993) 'Want do birthmothers want?' *Adoption and Fostering* 17 (4): 22–7.

Welshman, J. (1999) 'The social history of social history: the issue of the "problem family", 1940–70', *British Journal of Social Work* 29: 457–76.

West, P. (2002) 'The new Ireland kicks ass', *New Statesman*, 17 June: 20–2.

Westcott, H. L. (1991) *Institutional Abuse of Children: From Research to Policy. A Review*, London: NSPCC.

White, S. (1998a) 'Time, temporality and child welfare', *Time and Society* 7 (1): 55–74.

White, S. (1998b) 'Interdiscursivity and child welfare: the ascent and durability of psycho-legalism', *Sociological Review* 46 (2): 264–92.

189

Williams, C. (1999) 'Connecting anti-racist and anti-oppressive theory and practice: retrenchment or reappraisal?' *British Journal of Social Work* 29: 211–30.

Williams, C., Soydan, H. and Johnson, M. R. D. (eds) (1998) *Social Work and Minorities*, London: Routledge.

Williams, H. S. and Webb, A. Y. (1992) *Outcome Funding: a New Approach to Public Sector Grantmaking and Contracting*, New York: Rensselaerville Institute.

Williams, J. (2001) '1998 Human Rights Act: social work's new benchmark', *British Journal of Social Work* 31: 831–44.

Williams, P. J. (2002) 'Racial privacy', *Nation*, 17 June: 9.

Wilson, F. (1999) 'Cultural control within the virtual organization', *Sociological Review* 47 (4): 672–95.

Wilson, H. (2002) 'Brain science, early intervention and "at risk" families: implications for parents, professionals and social policy', *Social Policy and Society* 1 (3): 191–203.

Winchester, R. (2000a) 'Government review backs local authority control of adoption', *Community Care*, 13–19 July: 2–3.

Winchester, R. (2000b) 'Which way forward for adoption?' *Community Care*, 20–26 April: 10–11.

Winchester, R. (2001a) 'Up close and personal', *Community Care*, 29 March–4 April: 18–21.

Winchester, R. (2001b) 'Health and probation gain benefit of skills drain', *Community Care*, 26 April–2 May: 12–14.

Woodhead, M. (1990) 'Psychology and the cultural construction of children's needs' in A. James and A. Prout (eds) *Constructing and Reconstructing Childhood*, London: Falmer.

Woodroofe, K. (1962) *From Charity to Social Work*, London: Routledge.

Working Party on Catholic Education in a Multiracial, Multicultural Society (1984) *Learning from Diversity: a Challenge for Catholic Education*, London: Catholic Media Office.

Yeates, N. (1999) 'Social politics and policy in an era of globalization: critical reflections', *Social Policy and Administration* 33 (4): 372–93.

Young, H. (2000) 'Pious words that hide a double penalty for the poor', *Guardian*, 22 June.

Youth Justice Board (2001a) 'Home Secretary: speech on youth justice reforms', press release, 21 March.

Youth Justice Board (2001b) 'Twenty-two areas to receive Intensive Supervision and Surveillance Programmes (ISSPs)', press release, 21 March.

Youth Justice Board (2002a) 'Securicor STC Ltd chosen as preferred bidder for the new secure training centre', press release, 18 July.

Youth Justice Board (2002b) 'Youth offending falls after parenting programmes, research shows', press release, 9 July.

INDEX